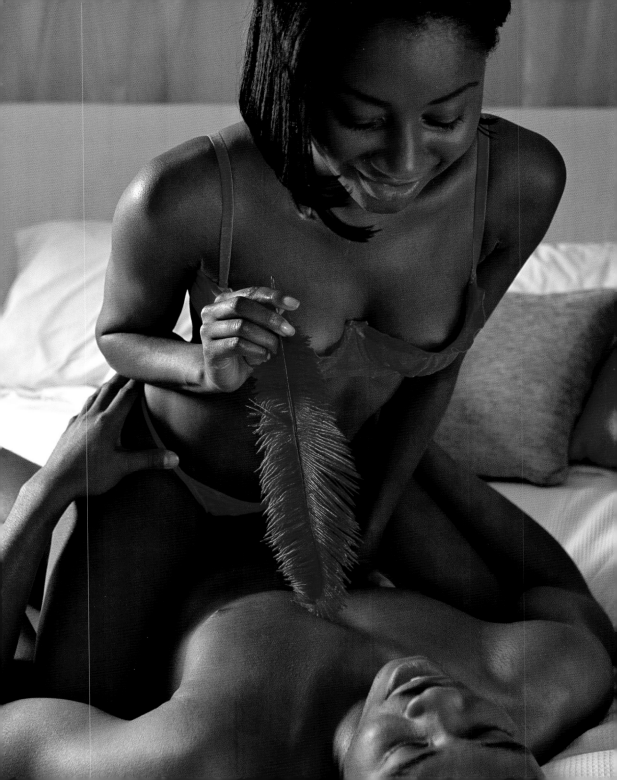

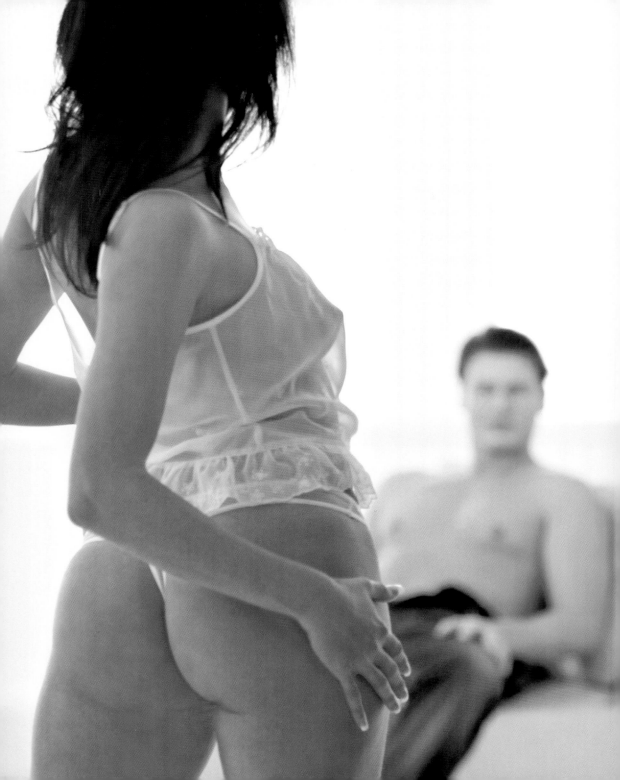

ANNE HOOPER

XXX SEX...
TONIGHT!

INTIMATE SEX SECRETS
TO KEEP HIM WANTING MORE

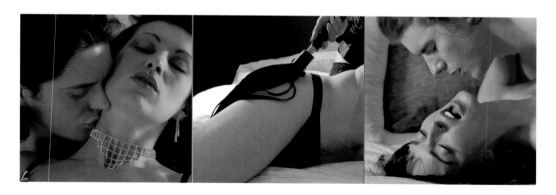

LONDON, NEW YORK, MUNICH,
MELBOURNE, DELHI

Brand Manager Lynne Brown
Senior Editor Jane Cooke
Senior Art Editor Helen Spencer
Project Art Editor Toni Kay
DTP Designer Traci Salter
Production Controllers Kevin Ward,
Mandy Inness
Photographer John Freeman
Stylist Claire Legemah
Publishing Director Corrine Roberts
Art Director Carole Ash

First published in the US in 2006
by DK Publishing Inc.,
375 Hudson Street, New York,
New York 10014

06 07 08 09 10 9 8 7 6 5 4 3 2 1

Cataloging-in-Publication data is
available from the Library of Congress

ISBN: 0-7566-1524-0
          978-0-75661-524-6

Color reproduction by Colourscan,
Singapore
Printed and bound by Star Standard,
Singapore

Discover more at:
www.dk.com

Contents

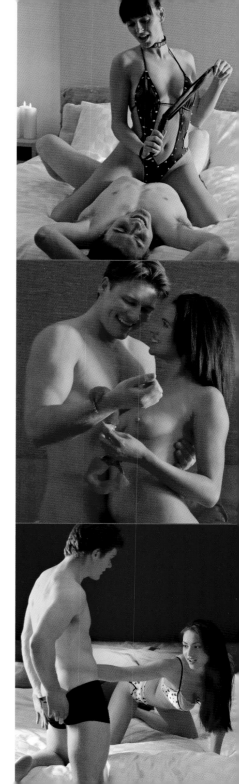

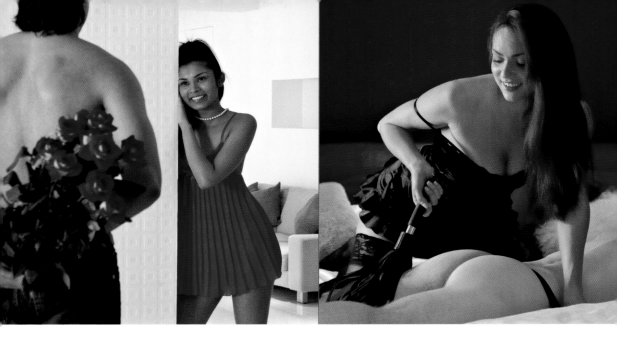

Introduction

Why do women want to please men, and why are men consistently receptive to female attention? You and your partner are alike in some ways, and yet fundamentally different in others. I think it's the differences between men and women that can make sex continually fascinating.

VENTURE INTO THE UNKNOWN

Exploring the differences between you and your man often seems like living on the edge. It entails a journey into the masculine unknown, which can feel uncomfortable but also potentially exciting. I believe that most women want to understand more about their partner's psyche and be able to connect with him on much deeper levels. Nowhere is the need for this understanding more apparent than in the bedroom.

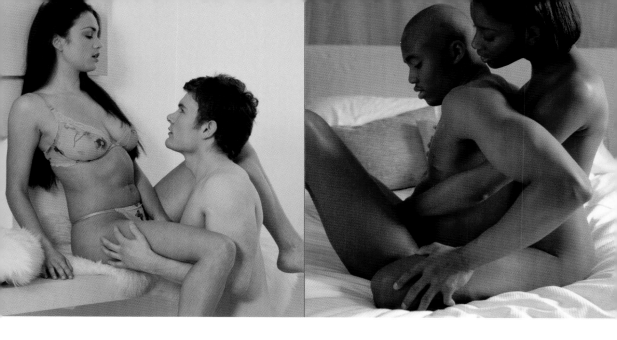

It's no coincidence that scores of men visit professional sex workers and, while we've been taught by society to regard this kind of sexual behavior as unsavory, we're prevented from understanding something valuable: however emotionally distant a sex worker is from her client she is clued into his urgent sexual desires. She will learn some very specific routes to the sexual pleasures that he really, really wants — and most sex workers will admit that these routes are not the ones he traverses at home.

ENTER MEN'S FANTASIES

Inhibition in both partners is an obvious hindrance to triple XXX sex. So, too, is the fear that if you disclose sexual secrets to someone intimate you expose yourself somehow to their power or you negatively alter the relationship. But I believe that it's possible to replace fear with energy and enthusiasm to achieve a far deeper intimacy. To help women enter the world of male fantasy, I've drawn on the experience of several "sex gurus" who know how this is best done — in my most x-rated book so far!

> " TRIPLE XXX SEX IS AN EXCITING ADVENTURE INTO THE UNKNOWN, WHICH CAN CONNECT YOU TO YOUR PARTNER ON A DEEP EMOTIONAL LEVEL. " *Anne*

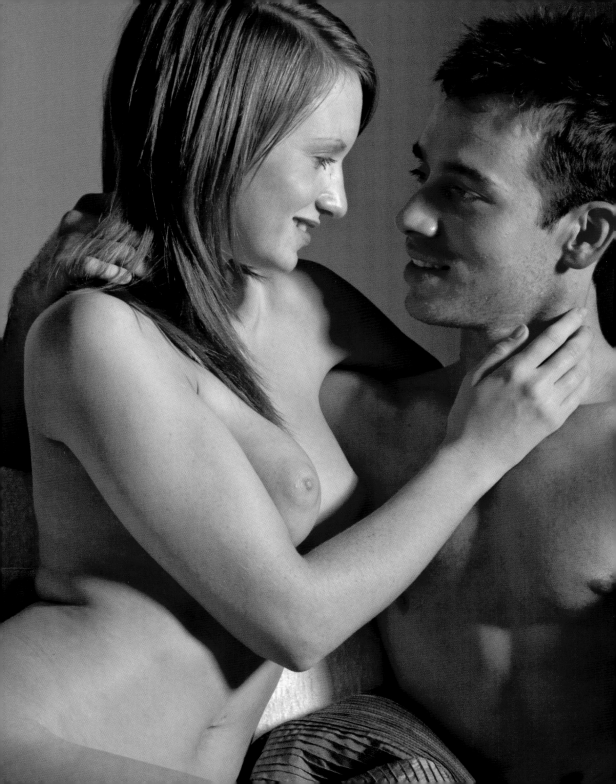

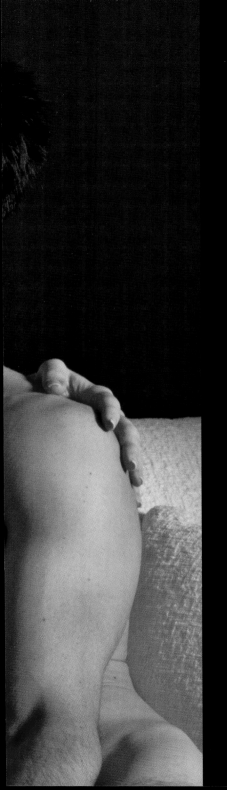

CHAPTER 1

Getting to know men

There has always been a tussle in the minds of men regarding their choice of partner. Should she be wife or mistress, Madonna or whore? And is it possible, or desirable, for one woman to be both? Your partner may enjoy being in charge of sex, or he may want to discover sex simultaneously with you. To get to know his innermost desires, take a look at the following pages and find out which kind of woman he desires and how you might match his ideal.

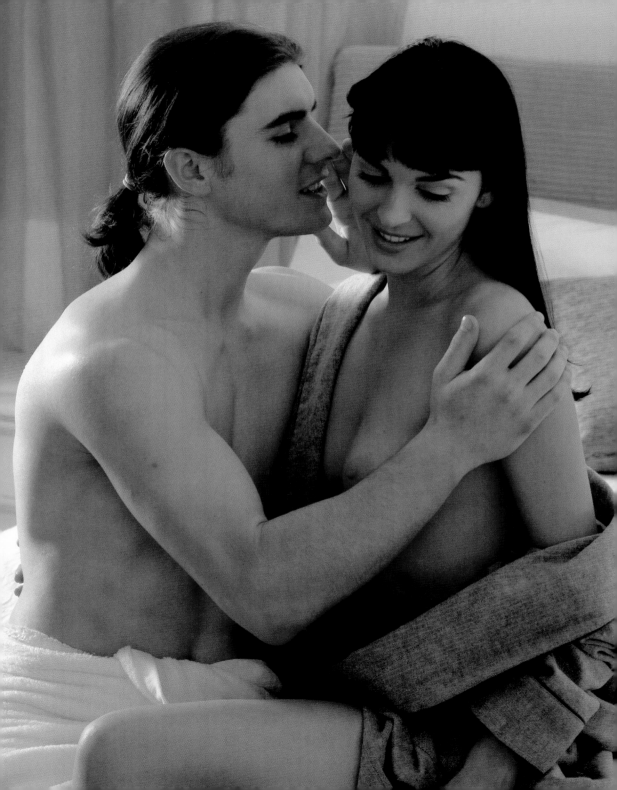

Men's secret desires

He may look the fresh-faced country boy, but are his innermost desires as innocent as his appearance? Here are three facts that highlight some realities about the male sex. I suggest you digest these before asking your partner the story of his life. Of course, *some* men are as open and honest as they look, but it's worth bearing in mind that others aren't!

THE **FACTS** OF **MEN**

1 Large numbers of married men go to hookers even though they are happily married.

2 Sex surveys show that men are not necessarily satisfied with the sex they have in their relationship in spite of loving their women.

3 Surveys of older people reveal that although they continue to consider themselves sexually active and experience orgasms regularly, much of this activity is not with their partner. Such men usually love their partners, however, and will stress the great affection they still have for their mate.

> " DIGGING DEEP INTO THE RECESSES OF HIS LUSTFUL IMAGINATION MAY SURPRISE OR AMUSE YOU. " *Anne*

WHAT'S YOUR **MAN'S** SEX **HISTORY?**

Is there a way of finding out what a partner really wants and then acting on it? If you're able to go that step further, will it keep a partner hot for you forever? Or might your exploratory frame of mind actually drive your man away? The best way of answering such questions is to take a kind of sex history — by simply talking to your man. This is much easier to do at the beginning of a relationship, but it's always possible even if it requires effort. The next pages contain the type of questions sex therapists ask when starting off with new clients.

TALKING TO MEN

Bombarding a brand new partner with questions may not be appropriate on first dates, but after a few meetings certain judiciously put questions can provide fascinating answers. Even if you don't see a major future with this person, it helps to know something about him. If there's a chance he is *the* man, then hearing some of the answers could be central to relationship success.

HOW TO ASK

The best way of asking questions is to let them pop out spontaneously. After sex is a good time or on a lazy "curled-up-on-the-sofa" occasion. You don't have to subject him to all your questions in one go. Just let the discussion evolve and continue it at a later date if necessary. Everyone likes others to be interested in them and most people enjoy talking about themselves given the opportunity.

You may have asked the following kind of questions intuitively without any prompting. These are my suggestions and you should, of course, word them in your own style. There may be some questions you can't bring yourself to ask. When this happens, ask yourself, "Is this my inhibition or am I picking up his?" The answer may be crucial. You could phrase your question like this: "There's something I've been wanting to know about you but I find it really difficult to ask. I'm not sure if this is my problem or something I'm picking up from you." Most human beings with an ounce of curiosity will immediately respond with, "What is it?" Over to you.

KEY QUESTIONS TO ASK HIM

1 What was your parents' background? How would you define their class, religion, and culture?

2 What were their moral attitudes and their views on play?

> " WHAT ARE HIS FANTASIES AND HOW CAN YOU ENTER THEM? YOU CAN'T TELL WHAT KIND OF A MAN YOURS IS UNTIL YOU DELVE DEEPER. " *Anne*

Sex secrets One of the mildest men I ever met turned out to be seriously into swinging, but he didn't dream of telling his wife because he was scared she'd be upset. Conversely, after tearing up the town, a tough biker I got to know used to serve amazing banquets to his partner prior to lovemaking.

3 What kind of "hidden" messages did you take in from your parents and how do you think they influenced you?

4 What are your earliest sexual memories? At what age did you start having wet dreams?

5 What is your earliest memory of sensual touch? (I mean innocent touch here.)

6 What were your earliest sexual thoughts and dreams?

7 What did you learn about sex from your friends at school?

8 When did you first masturbate and what was your reaction the first few times?

9 When did you first have sexual fantasies and can you remember any of them?

10 When did you first get interested in a girl?

11 Did you ever get interested in a boy?

12 What was your first experience of intercourse?

13 Did you ever suffer any humiliating sexual experiences?

14 On what occasion did sex go really well? What were the potent ingredients?

15 What kind of sex would you like to experience, given absolute freedom?

16 What are your adult fantasies and would you like them to become reality?

17 How might a partner fit into your fantasies?

18 How have your sexual relationships gone in the past?

Anne's advice

Comparing sexual backgrounds gives you some idea of how similar or different your experiences are. This gives you some good pointers about the direction in which your man might want to travel. You can then ask yourself "Is this what I want?" If his sexual interests go too far for you it might well be the time to tactfully bow out of the relationship.

HOW TO USE HIS ANSWERS

There are no right answers to any of the above – just information that you can use to form a clearer picture of your man's sexual psyche. You're trying to put together a picture of his emotional and sexual development, which is why you're trying to take an informal sexual history. It ought to go without saying that for a relationship to go really well, your man needs to be interested in a similar conversation about you.

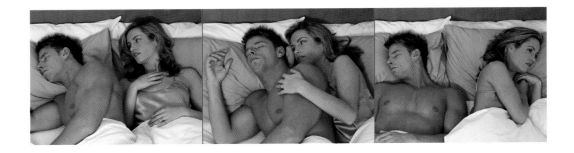

What men want —
and women don't

The way men express themselves sexually often requires some clever female interpretation. Here are some common differences in behavior that can adversely affect your sex life if you can't read the signs.

HE CAN'T SAY HE **LOVES YOU** BUT HE **ALWAYS WANTS SEX** WITH YOU

Underneath this overactive behavior is an anxious man. He's anxious to feel that you love him, but he's confused love with physical expression. The man who says, "Of course I love you, I screw you, don't I?" isn't being coarse. He's saying that his way of showing love relies on sexual behavior rather than speech.

He may have come from a tough background where he was taught to suppress emotion. For him revealing love means being vulnerable, but wanting sex is OK because it's manly. And so the two get confused – he uses sex for love. Your response might be, "I do believe you love me, but just as you need a lot of sex, I need to hear the words 'I love you' occasionally."

HE GETS **HORNY** IN THE **MIDDLE** OF AN **ARGUMENT**

Sex is the last thing on your mind after a quarrel and yet he's the one to feel hurt when you push him away in bed. This guy may be adrenalized by the argument and he mistakes physical arousal for sexual excitement, as some women do. But the man who rapidly reacts like this may be feeling nervous underneath his macho exterior. A quarrel puts him in touch with fear, and in his mind the best method of reassurance is to get as close to you physically as he can — sex, of course, being the ultimate in physical closeness.

Your best bet is to stay cool but explain your view. You might say, "I think we both need to calm down and then I might well want to have sex." If you can manage this, you're letting him know that although you're in a different frame of mind sexually, you will desire him again in the future.

HE SOMETIMES **WANTS SEX** WITHOUT **MAKING LOVE**

You've discovered in the mornings that although your man seems to start off wanting sex with you, he will apparently change his mind, get short-tempered and leap out of bed. When you ask him what the matter is, he explains that he really feels like quick, mindless sex and not like spending a long time on foreplay. Because he thought you'd never stand for this, he backs off before things go too far. And he feels extremely grumpy as a result.

Are men right to think such sexual activity would be totally unacceptable? Or can it be accommodated in a flexible relationship? There are many different sexual experiences to enjoy within one relationship — quick, lusty sex is included. This type of sex might be considered wrong if it were the sole way in which your man ever wanted to have sex with you. But you might feel perfectly comfortable agreeing that sometimes sex should be just for him.

" THANKS TO SEX PROFESSIONALS LIKE XAVIERA HOLLANDER, WE KNOW HOW MUCH MEN VALUE WOMEN WHO PAY ATTENTION TO THE WAY THEY THINK. " *Anne*

Anne's advice When you get to know men better, it becomes clear that their sexual expressions cry out for correct interpretation by women. By successfully interpreting male behavior (if you can gauge the thoughts behind your partner's actions), your reaction to it may be more positive.

HE WANTS **SEX** AFTER YOU'VE HAD AN **EXHAUSTING** DAY **CARING** FOR THE **BABY**

This man believes that you're giving all your attention to the baby. He fears that there's no attention left over for him. He needs reassurance at this tricky emotional time and to know that you still love him at least as much as you love the baby. So, he pressures for attention by demanding sex.

I would never encourage a woman to make love when it's the last thing she feels like, but I do believe in offering reassurance. You might say, "I absolutely adore you darling. You are the light of my life. Let me go and put the baby down so that I can hold you." Hold him close but explain, when he wants to go further, that a warm embrace is the sexiest experience for you at the moment. But keep holding him and keep telling him how much you love and appreciate him. It's reassurance you're giving here rather than sex.

HE **ALWAYS** WANTS **SEX** IN **EXACTLY** THE SAME **ROUTINE**

Not all men want sex in a variety of ways. Some guys, having hit on a successful sex pattern, seem incapable of stepping outside it. If you ask them to budge on their loving moves – even an inch – they react as if you've offered the worst kind of criticism. As far as they're concerned, there's a right way and a wrong way to do sex and that's all there is to it! This can be frustrating to an exploratory lover who may long for change.

I've found by observing my therapy clients that the best way to appeal to this sort of man is to focus on his personal system of logic. Is it a question of right and wrong to him? Does he fear doing something new? Can you help him by offering him a system of graduated steps toward changing his sexual moves? If you can encourage him to see change as a pattern, there's a greater chance of adjustment.

Anne's advice There is a tendency for women to hold back from fully entering the male mindset. This could be because we're afraid of potentially unpalatable male desires, or that male demands might leave our own needs out of the equation. But once we can interpret male desires and their meaning, perhaps our reaction to them changes.

" THE SMALLEST INITIAL CHANGE TO YOUR SEX ROUTINE CAN SOW THE SEEDS FOR GREATER CHANGE IN HIS MIND. " *Anne*

HE **WITHDRAWS EMOTIONALLY** AFTER **SEX.** WHY?

Your man is with you all the way– relating to you utterly through the waves of sexual excitement as he talks, jokes, strokes, and caresses. He seems to be the perfect lover until…after the big event. Once the orgasms are over he becomes a different man. He moves away, won't or can't talk, and isn't interested in snuggling. You feel rejected because this seems so wrong. Is it something you did or is he feeling separated from you?

This could be an extreme physical reaction to the sexual experience. He's put out so much energy and feeling that he literally has to recharge his batteries. When someone's completely drained, it's very hard to even move. After orgasm it's normal to be flooded with relaxing feelings and this is a key time to drift off into a doze.

There is another explanation of such behavior. My own psychological theory is that many men feel they must be in control. They do, of course, lose their control at the moment of orgasm — they can't help it — and their subsequent withdrawal is about regaining control.

Anne's advice Your best method for coping with emotional withdrawal – or worse, sleeping – after sex is to understand his needs and try to tolerate them. When you're not making love, you could let him know that a post-coital snuggle is important to you while he goes through his recovery.

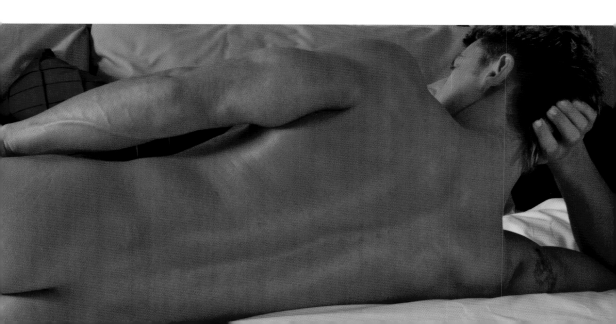

Male turn ons

Once you've got to know and appreciate your man's sexual psyche, you can choose which of the following seduction scenarios (here and on the following pages) will appeal to him the most. The chances are that all five of them will have him begging for more of you.

SHE HAS NO **INHIBITIONS** OR **HANG UPS**

She's someone who is completely at home in her own body and in her man's. She doesn't mind getting into his intimate body crevices, nor does she have a problem exploring the more sophisticated variations of sex. It helps if she's highly orgasmic but this isn't a must. What really counts is the way she impales herself on her man's erections, the eagerness with which she discovers his prostate gland, and the delight in which she joins in with games of mild submission and domination. There's no need to feel guilty or ashamed with this woman because she never does.

> " UNLESS SEDUCTION MOVES SUIT MEN AS INDIVIDUALS, THEY JUST FEEL LIKE PERFORMANCES PUT ON BY WOMEN. "
> *Anne*

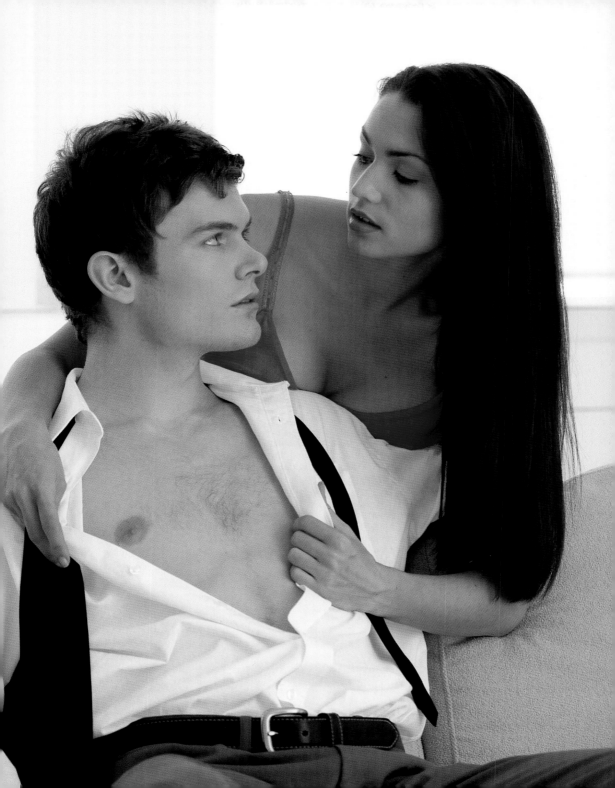

SHE CAN'T GET **ENOUGH** OF **HIM**

Her enthusiasm carries the day. The fact that she can't get enough of her partner is immensely flattering to him. Her obvious adoration (she finds every sexual move he makes massively erotic) is a huge turn on. This woman has no problems with frequency because her man has a devastating effect on her. Not for her the actions of making love out of habit or duty. This woman wants her man, she wants all of him, and she shows it very clearly.

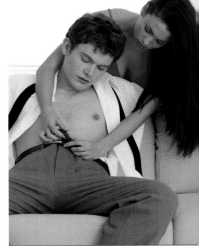

SHE'S **SEXUALLY** SOPHISTICATED

This is the female with *Kama Sutra* expertize. She's every man's fantasy of the slightly older French woman who initiates the innocent lad into pleasures previously undreamed of. She is a lady of experience who understands how her body works and, more importantly, how the male body works too. She teaches by example, so when he feels unable to stop himself from climaxing, oh joy, she takes control and suddenly he can last for hours. Because she has learned sexual techniques, she uses her knowledge to make the right moves.

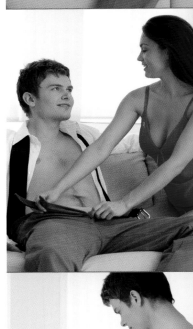

SHE TAKES THE **SEXUAL INITIATIVE**

She doesn't wait for the man to make a move – she starts right on in. If you knew how men long to have some of the responsibility for sex taken off their shoulders, you wouldn't hesitate here. I'm not talking about steamrollering your man, but I am suggesting that you should initiate and then wait for a response. Then you should follow up that response with further action before taking another sounding. Good sex is about reciprocation; wonderful, spontaneous sex flows out of the two of you and is truly creative.

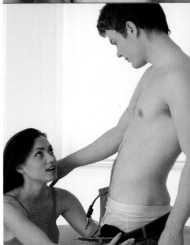

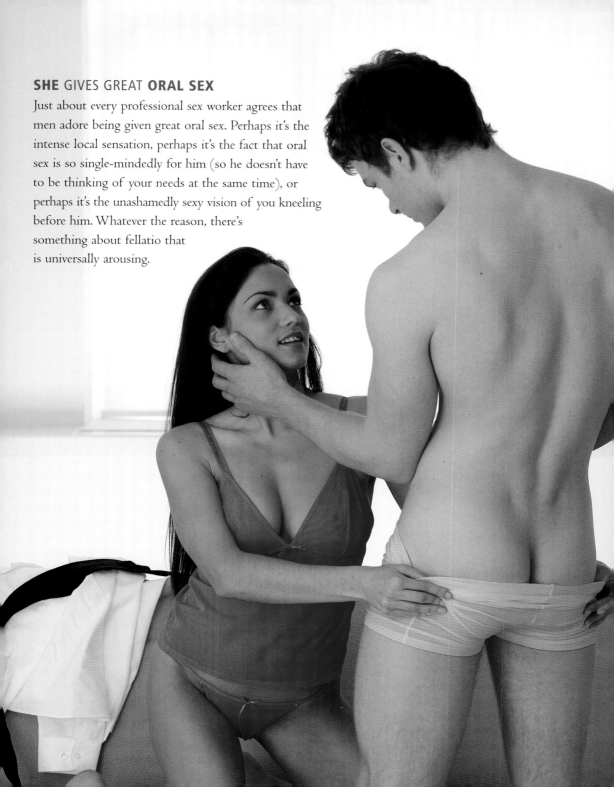

SHE GIVES GREAT ORAL SEX

Just about every professional sex worker agrees that
men adore being given great oral sex. Perhaps it's the
intense local sensation, perhaps it's the fact that oral
sex is so single-mindedly for him (so he doesn't have
to be thinking of your needs at the same time), or
perhaps it's the unashamedly sexy vision of you kneeling
before him. Whatever the reason, there's
something about fellatio that
is universally arousing.

Male turn offs

We hear a lot about how easily men are turned on, but not so much about what turns them off, which can be just as important. I carried out a straw poll of my male friends and relations and they all agreed on the following three very definite "no-nos" regarding the opposite sex.

WOMEN WHO CRITICIZE

Most men long for their women to admire them and praise them to the skies. They want to be made to feel wonderful — in spite of knowing that many of their actions are far from wonderful. In fact, men hate being criticized. The more you criticize, the greater his sense of a knife being twisted in his vitals! So should you ever criticize? Aren't there times when you think the entire future of the sexual relationship depends on you speaking up?

There's a huge difference between destructive and constructive criticism. Criticism that is constant, harping, and accusatory undermines any person's pride and self-confidence and results in very little except pain and anger. If someone tells you that you are terrible at oral sex, for example, you feel awful and have little incentive to ever do it again. Men are easily overwhelmed by a woman's criticism, to an extent that their entire sexual performance can be destabilized.

Much less harmful is constructive criticism. This consists of comment tempered by praise. For example, "I'm overjoyed you want to go down on me. I particularly like it when you use your tongue to stroke my clitoris upwards — it feels amazing. Please could you do tons more of it?" You've made him feel great while asking him to do something extra to please you.

Sex secrets Xaviera Hollander, formerly New York's "most successful madam" taught what she called her first principle of sex: that you should make your man feel like a god if you want to be the sex goddess of his dreams.

WOMEN WHO **SMELL** STRONG

Men can find strong perfume so overpowering that it forms a barrier. Contrary to what many women believe, men don't go for very strong scents because the male nose scents us more delicately than we do ourselves. What may seem like a dash of perfume or the scent of intimacy to the innocent female, can be overwhelming to her man.

Dab perfume on certain spots, rather than spraying it all over, and go for light flowery fragrances rather than the heavy musky ones. Don't try to hide your natural bodily scents under the arms and around the vagina. These are sexy smells and not repellent unless you have an infection or don't wash thoroughly and regularly.

Sex secrets Emperor Napoleon Bonaparte's famous command when returning home to his wife Josephine was, "I'm coming home. Don't wash." The great man found the natural earthy smells of his wife powerfully erotic.

WOMEN WHO ARE **SQUEAMISH**

The trouble with a squeamish woman is that she can make her man feel bad for wanting something perfectly sexually normal. Of course, some men are squeamish too and would reject an anal massage faster than you could say "orgasm." But some men adore the idea of getting really hot, sweaty, smelly, and snuggled into unexplored regions and they feel frustrated when they meet with a scream of disgust – it's a recipe for dissatisfaction.

Women who are squeamish run the risk of not just annoying their men, but of missing out on some wonderful sexual experiences. Germaine Greer wrote in 1968, "If you've never tasted your own menstrual blood sister, you haven't lived." This sentence horrified a generation of women, but it made them think. They expected their men to be comfortable tasting their vaginal juices, so didn't it make sense to be comfortable about them themselves? And didn't it also mean that women should be a lot more comfortable with their man's most intimate areas, tastes, and smells as well?

" MEN FEEL MORE SEXUALLY AT EASE WITH WOMEN WHO ARE COMFORTABLE WITH THEIR BODIES AND BODILY FUNCTIONS. "
Anne

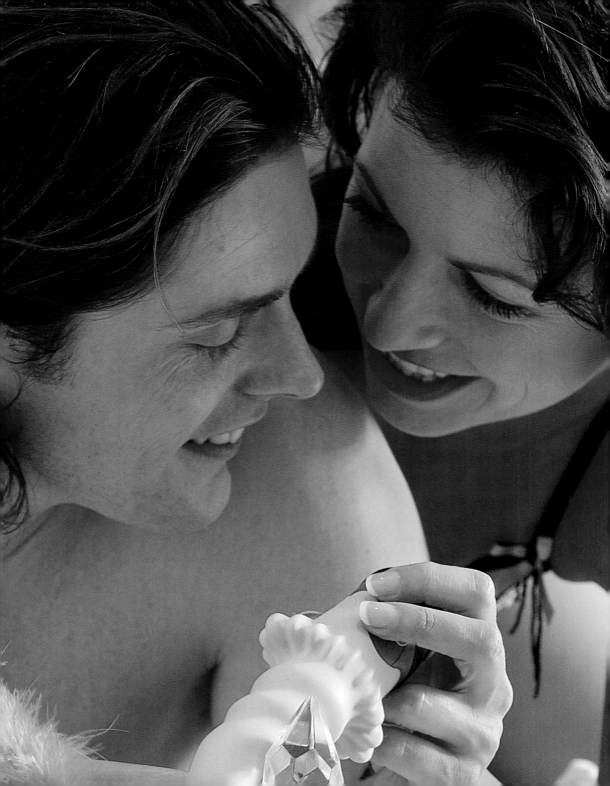

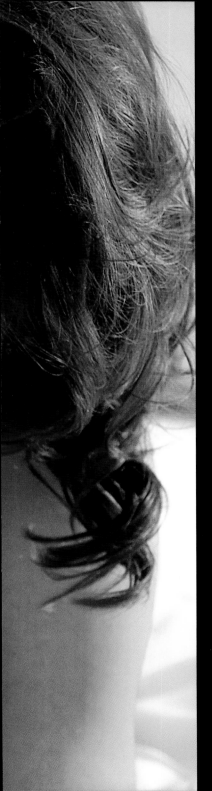

CHAPTER 2

Triple XXX mindset

One of the keys to becoming your man's greatest lover is to gauge what it's like to be male. What might the physical feelings be and, given free choice, how might your emotional behavior differ as a male? Once you have some insight into the sexual depths of his soul, then comes the time to understand your own state of mind. By exploring your sexual psyche, you can develop the confidence to arouse him more, drive him harder, and ultimately overwhelm his mind and body.

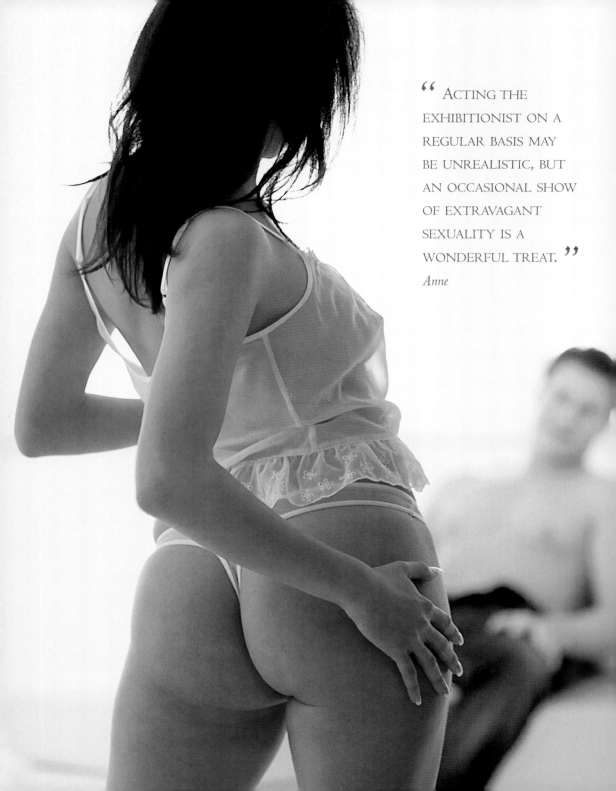

Encourage your inner exhibitionist

Many women find it hard to "show off" in front of their man and yet many men adore being a voyeur. These are men who long to watch you perform striptease, masturbate, or be extravagantly sexual. Men are turned on by what they see far more than women are. It's one of the proven sex differences, and if you want to wow your guy you could hardly do better than work out the best way to give him a good show.

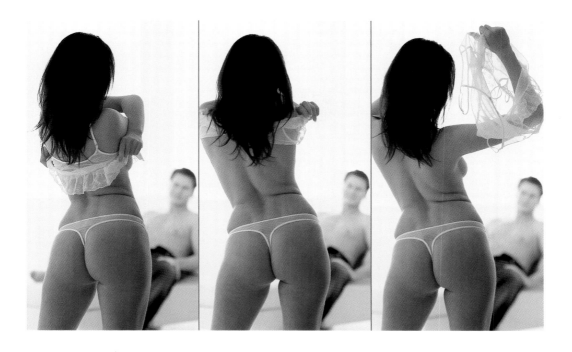

EXHIBITIONIST ROUTINE

- **Undress** in front of a tall mirror and, taking it slowly, pull off each garment deliberately.
- **Examine** your body and caress it.
- **Dance** provocatively for your personal pleasure only. If you feel silly, simply slowly and sensuously bend your body from side to side and roll your hips. It certainly helps to do this to some sexy music.
- **Sit down** (still naked) in a big armchair in front of the mirror and begin touching your body and genitals, slipping yourself surreptitious glances from time to time.

Anne's advice Build on the sexual feelings you experience as they grow and let yourself go with the sensations. You're not trying for orgasm, but aiming to enjoy pure sensation for its own sake.

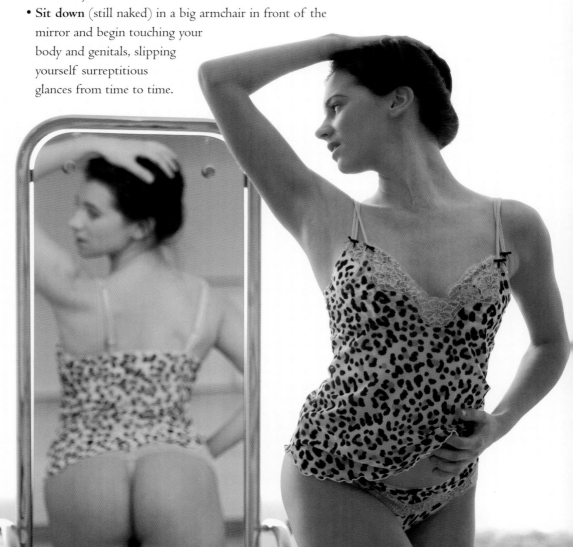

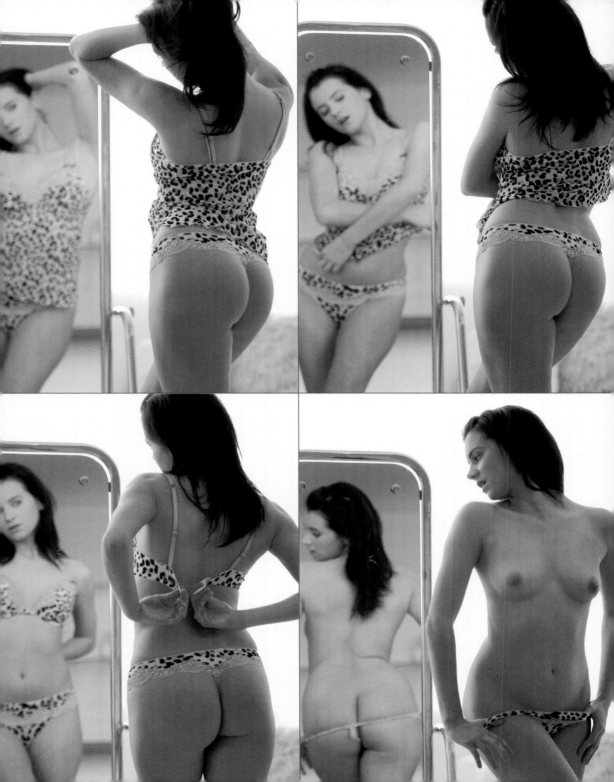

Explore your fantasies

According to John Bancroft, former director of the Kinsey Institute, testosterone stimulates the sexual imagination. If so, this probably explains why many men are more prone to sexual fantasy than women. Since fantasy can be an important facet of sexuality, it's a good idea to get a handle on what your man might be inwardly yearning for. But first you need to explore your own fantasies and get comfortable with them.

LEARNING TO FANTASIZE

A fantasy can help build up sexual stimulation so effectively that it seriously heightens your climax. For women with difficulty climaxing, a fantasy can develop sexual arousal sufficiently for orgasm to be experienced for the first time.

But a great many women aren't comfortable with sexual fantasy and devise justifications for keeping their minds "pure" during sex. These justifications may be part of a defense system to combat feelings of failure should sexual fantasy prove difficult to experience. My clinical work has shown that some women find the use of sexual fantasy difficult, others impossible, and even those women who fantasize often and imaginatively tend not to have such "hard core" sexual imaginations as many men.

If yours is the kind of brain that automatically thinks of the day in the office or the children or housework, you may find it difficult to switch over to something more ethereal. If you haven't fantasized naturally, the odds are you need something to help you kick-start the blue movies in your mind. A few moments of peace in a sensual environment with some sexy literature for inspiration may be all you need.

Stress-relax exercise

Start with your toes and then work your way slowly up the rest of your body. Tense the toes for a count of three then relax them. You'll find that if you do the same tense-and-relax sequence right up to the face and head, your entire body will become relaxed. If parts of your body remain tense, go back to those parts and repeat the exercise.

FANTASY STEPS

1 The first step when learning to fantasize is to find quiet, private space for yourself. Unplug the phone, lock the bedroom door, and ensure that there'll be no interruptions. If necessary hang a notice on the door. Do whatever is likely to de-stress you. My suggestions include taking a warm bath with scented oils, simply lying in your heated bedroom with sweet smells and soft music playing, or trying the stress-relax exercise opposite.

2 Let your mind roam until a sexy thought or idea comes into your brain. Don't brush it away but explore it further. Let the fantasy unfold naturally – if it helps, begin to stimulate yourself at the same time. During the course of the week, you can go back to the fantasy and enlarge or extend it. Take your fantasy a little bit further each time you recall it and take it as far as you can.

3 If a sexy thought refuses to appear in your brain, sexy books can be a genuine help. Some women like soft-core photos, while many prefer sexy literature. One tried and tested erotic book is *My Secret Garden*, a collection of women's fantasies by Nancy Friday (see also p.214).

4 Think about writing down your fantasy, asking your man to do the same with his, and then sharing both sets of fantasies together. By exploring your sexual imagination and being unafraid to share it, you could open up a completely new aspect of your joint sexuality.

5 Find a volume of men's fantasies and read it carefully. Ask yourself if you feel you can understand and accept what you read. Recommended reads are *Men in Love* by Nancy Friday, and *My Secret Garden Shed*, edited by Paul Scott.

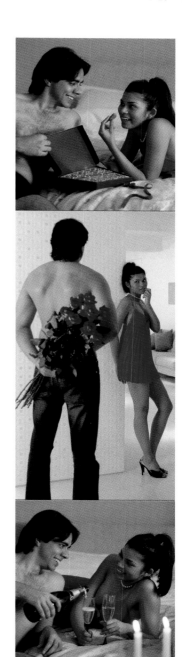

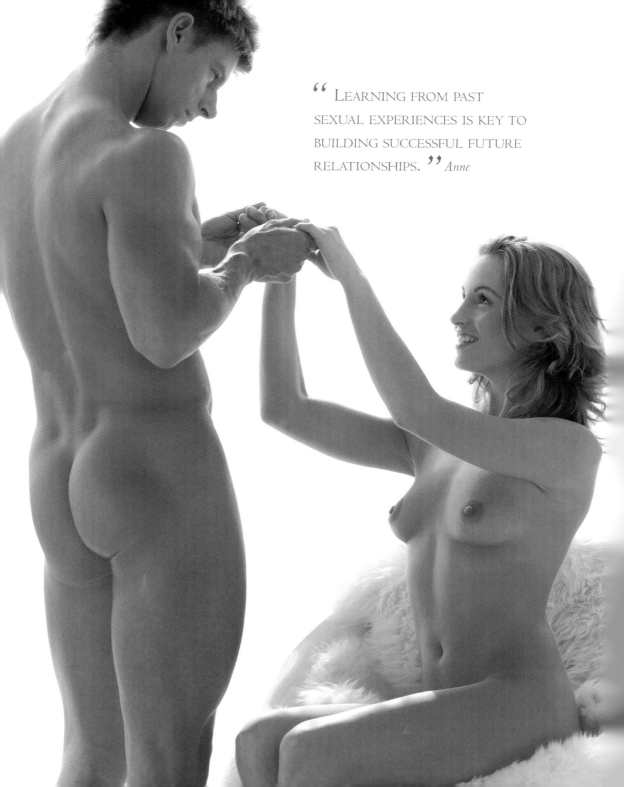

Build on experience

Learning to be a good lover and to select a good lover stems, to an extent, from past judgments and experiences. Through these you build up a mental reference library and learn to recognize the "signs," or invisible psychological clues, about a man's potential. Hopefully, you use this library to adjust your choices in successive relationships, so that you end up with someone better suited to the sensual gifts you wish to bestow.

YOUR **BEST** AND **WORST EXPERIENCES**

Think about your best sexual experiences in the unheated calm of your mind when you're not actually in the throes of lovemaking. Does your experience tell you what really works for you? You could try this imagining that you are your lover. Can you get a handle on what works for him this way, and do your experiences marry up? If not, what might you be able to change?

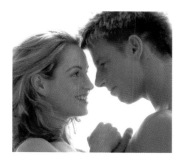

Bernie Zilbergeld (see p.219), a US therapist and leading expert specializing in male sexual problems, suggests you think of your three best sexual experiences then write down the powerful ingredients of these scenarios as a reminder of what was so great. Try to imagine at least one experience if you can't remember three.

The details of your experience could be quite mundane, like the warmth of the bedroom or the lighting in the room, or quite extreme, like when you almost fainted the first time you had an orgasm. Zilbergeld also suggests that you should write down your three worst sexual experiences and think about how they might have been more positive in light of your "best experience" findings.

Anne's advice I will add to Zilbergeld's exercises by suggesting you ask your lover to list his best and worst sexual experiences. If he is willing to share these experiences, you may learn much about each other. This isn't a competition but simply an opportunity for you both to put your past sexual experiences into perspective.

What sex are you?
What sex is he?

Think before you claim unequivocally to be either one sex or the other. Each of us possesses both masculine and feminine qualities that affect our entire being, including our sexuality. Masculinity and femininity are derived from our genetic make-up, the conditions we encounter in the womb, and what we learn from our surroundings once born. All three of these interrelate, so try to see your man as a challenge to unravel.

THE **INDEX-FINGER** TEST

Do want to find out the extent of your man's sexual potential without him having a clue about your sleuthing? Here's how. The relative lengths of your index and ring fingers (your second and fourth digits) are partly determined by the levels of sex hormones your body produces. Men who produce lots of testosterone generally have longer ring fingers relative to their index fingers. Women who produce high levels of female sex hormones (including oestrogen, prolactin, and luteinizing hormone) generally have shorter ring fingers relative to their index fingers.

With this in mind, take look at his hands and do a spot of surreptitious measuring. You should be able to judge this by eye. If your man has relatively short ring fingers, he may be a lot gentler than he appears on the surface. And if you have relatively long ring fingers this may mean that, despite your fluttery femininity, you are highly sexed, confident, and waiting for the opportunity to explore your sexuality further.

" WE ALL HAVE DIFFERING COMBINATIONS OF MASCULINE AND FEMININE QUALITIES THAT PROFOUNDLY AFFECT OUR SEX LIVES. " *Anne*

Fact check Testosterone is a male sex hormone produced by the testes and by the ovaries in very small amounts. As well as stimulating sex organ development, it progresses muscle growth.

THE **HAIR** TESTS

Testosterone affects male hair patterns on the head. He may look like an Adonis in his 20s, but he may rapidly lose his locks in his 30s and eventually go bald. The upside of this is that he's likely to be full of energy and enthusiasm, not to mention easily sexually aroused. One way of finding out how your Adonis may end up is by taking a look at his father – baldness usually runs in the family.

As a general rule, women with a lot of body hair and slight acne are likely to possess high levels of testosterone. This not only means that they may enjoy an easier sexual response but it also affects their energy, strength, and possibly their sexual imagination. These women may be a sexual dream, but their partners need to know they can cope with the accompanying assertiveness.

HOW DO YOU **FEEL – MASCULINE** OR **FEMININE?**

There are no standard answers to this question. It took me years to realize that my feelings were a combination of rather passive femininity (I love it when my man makes the moves) plus some surprisingly masculine traits. I really liked taking the initiative as long as my lover accepted this completely. The minute he resisted, I closed down and became passive again. My natural sexual energy had a powerful outer layer of "feminine" conditioning. If you are lucky enough to find a partner with whom you can talk freely, this sort of shared information is both exciting and enlightening.

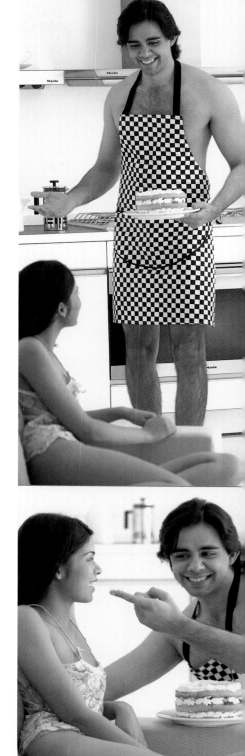

Cycles of great sex

It's common knowledge that an attractive lover has an overpowering effect on us, literally making us "hot" with desire. But you may not be aware of sex cycles, which are times in our lives or in the year when we're more likely to become hot. Both sexes are subject to these cycles, explained overleaf. Take the case of a woman who is attracted to man. The attraction may be oneway to start with, but the fact that she's hot for him makes her more attractive. Similarly, the man who's hot acts as a honeypot to various female "bees."

" THE SECRET IS TO PREDICT THE TIME IN A SEX CYCLE WHEN YOU'RE MOST LIKELY TO SPONTANEOUSLY COMBUST. " *Anne*

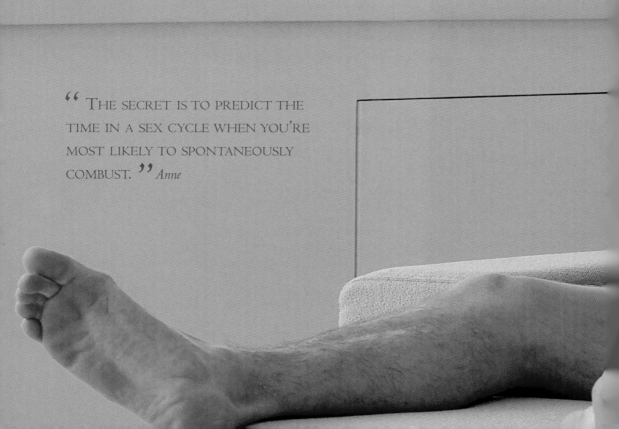

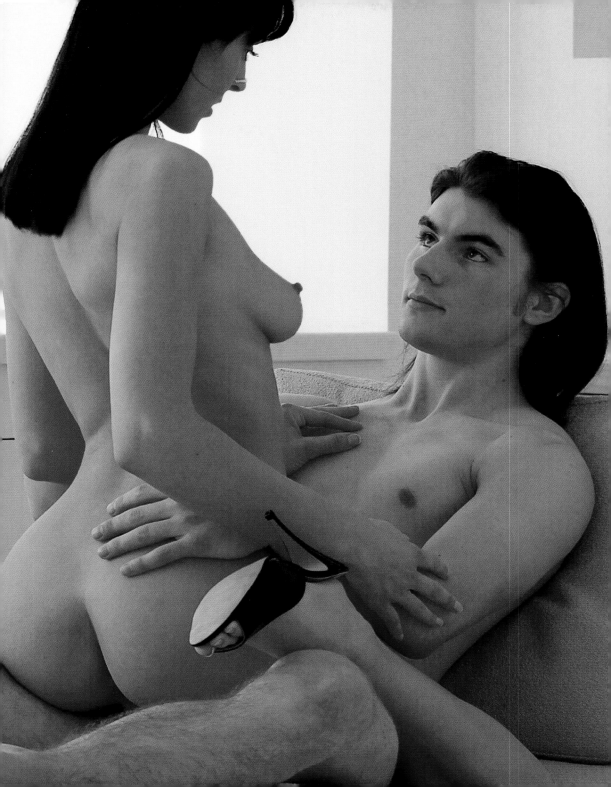

CYCLES OF ATTRACTION

Sex educators, Steve and Vera Bodansky (see p.218), recognize a cycle of attraction that results from a physical or geographical situation. They cite the phenomenon of a man moving into some kind of shared house or community where many of the women are simultaneously attracted to him and subsequently make a play. (I've seen this happen at conferences.) The guy thinks he's died and gone to heaven, of course. After a few months, during which several woman pursue him, most of them lose interest and he ends up with one permanent partner.

The growing belief behind this course of events is that a substance in a man's sweat is a powerful sexual attractant to new women around him. When men feel particularly sexy, perhaps because they're in contact with new women or in a new sexual relationship, they mysteriously become extra attractive to other women as well as their partners.

MENSTRUAL CYCLES

Each menstrual cycle last for roughly 28 days, during which time female hormone levels rise and fall in a predictable pattern. What's less well known is that with this hormonal fluctuation goes a corresponding fluctuation in sexual desire.

There are two recognized high points in this cycle of sexual desire. The first is the time around ovulation (roughly the middle of the menstrual month) and the second, much more powerful point in my opinion, is right at the end of the menstrual cycle when sexual sensitivity rises sky high and some women only have to be touched to feel amazing.

This extra-sensual time results from the fact that both estrogen and progesterone hormone levels are down, leaving more hormonal receptors available for testosterone, which is the hormone responsible for sex drive. You may also give off a more musky smell than usual, which is likely to be a powerful

Anne's advice

Remember this cycle of attraction next time you change your physical surroundings. You might, for example, take a new job and move to a new workplace. Newcomers have a subtle effect on the men and women they come into contact with and it's a good time to make a play!

Research check

Dr. Glenn Wilson in *Love's Mysteries* (1976) refers to several studies showing that men are attracted to women who are turned on by the scent of their sweat.

subliminal attractant. Predicting your secret monthly "windows" can result in some incredible sex. You might bear these special times in mind when planning dates or romantic breaks in advance.

SEASONAL CYCLES

The great majority of us live in cities and are therefore less subject to the variations of weather and temperature. Nevertheless, even city dwellers recognize the fact that it tends to be hot in summer and cold in winter. Extreme heat and cold are both unsympathetic to the libido, using up energy and forcing us to conserve what's left rather than use it in brisk movement and easy sexual expression.

Spring and fall, however, are well recognized as seasons of renewal and consolidation. These are the times of year when temperatures enable us to regain energy and general perkiness. These are the times of year when marriages are made and babies conceived.

Anne's advice If you want to ensure a period of maximum sexiness, arrange a liaison in spring or fall that coincides with the second half of your menstrual period.

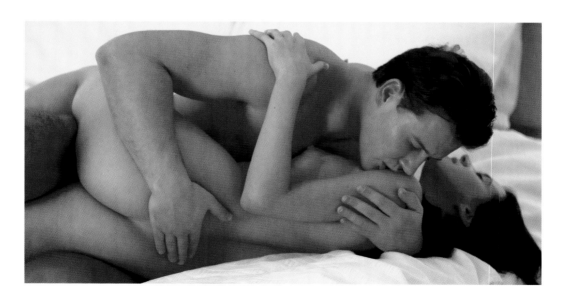

Box of sex secrets

Turn yourself on by preparing a sexual box of tricks. You'll certainly stimulate your man's curiosity and generate apprehension if you show it off to him. Sex professional, Xaviera Hollander (see p.218), recommends putting together what she calls a "fun box." Her fun box includes a library of erotica that you can read out loud with your partner, along with some seriously raunchy pictures.

ANNE HOOPER'S **FUN BOX**

The assembling of my fun box starts off with consideration of the exterior. A sleazy cardboard container with some worn-out dildos spilling out at the edge isn't going to cause much delightful anticipation of the contents. My ideal kind of toy chest needs to look either smart or artistically sexy. Since you're unlikely to find a "sex box supplier" very easily, you'll need to think creatively. Plain, but beautifully-finished black or red lacquer on the outside of the box is both discreet and attractive, for example, as is a covering of bold pink silk. The inside might be padded with a wispy chiffon or a gleaming satin.

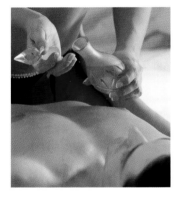

A friend of mine pasted wonderful art nouveau drawings on the outside of her box and then sealed it with a transparent lacquer. The drawings depicted willowy females partly draped in transparent muslins and partly draped in each other.

Since you won't want any passing browsers to delve into the mysteries of your coffer uninvited, put a padlock on it. A beautiful silver or gold one will add to the intrigue.

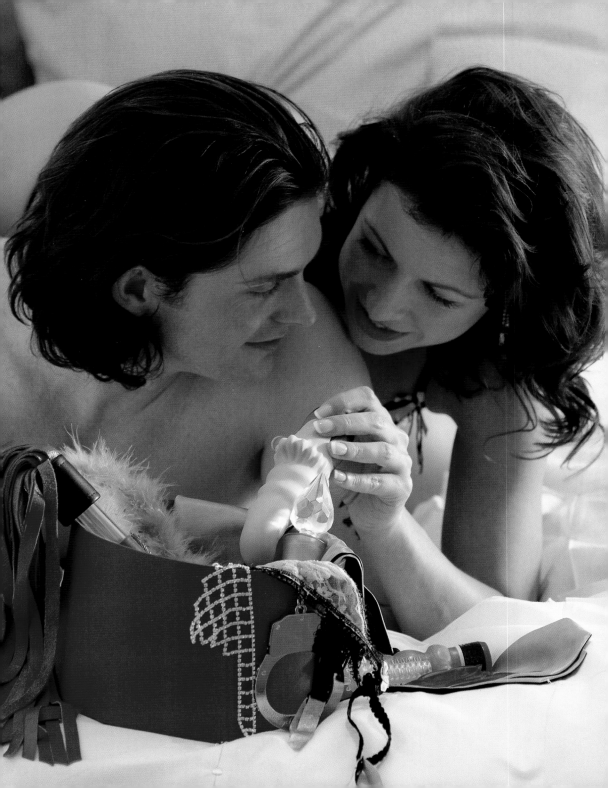

SECRET TREASURES

1 Jewelry

2 Souvenirs – you might exchange intimate sets of underwear with a lover

3 A goody bag – containing handcuffs, self-adhesive tattoos, a black blindfold, a suspender belt, a kinky heart-shaped bottom paddle or fur collar and lead

4 Favorite vibrator

5 Lubes – perhaps the tasteless, odorless, nongreasy lubricants that mimic your natural juices, or the gel-filled ones for oral sex

6 Pictures and photographs

7 Massage oil in a beautiful glass bottle

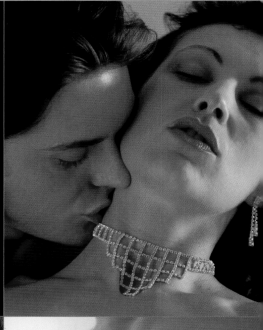

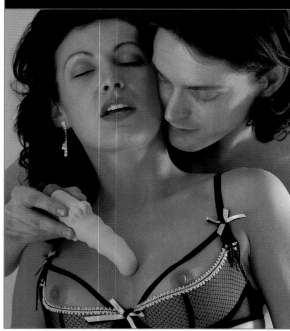

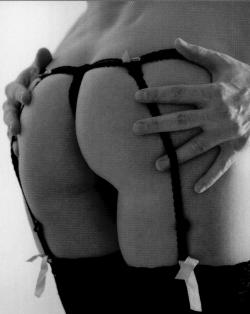

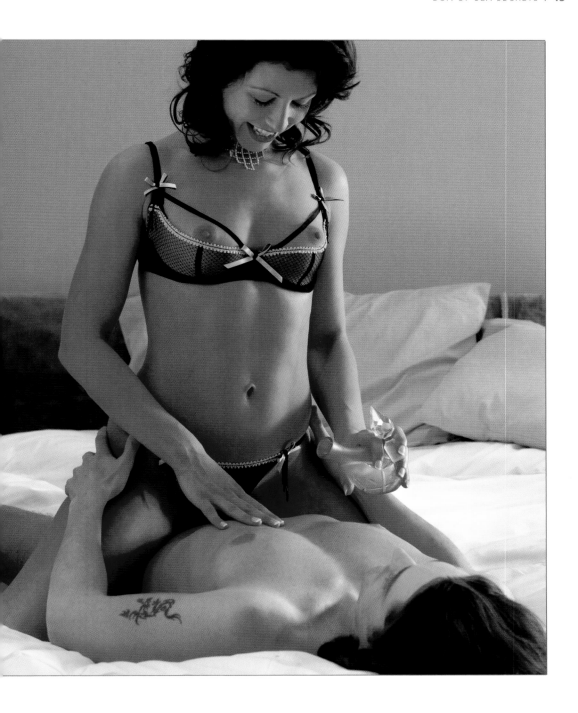

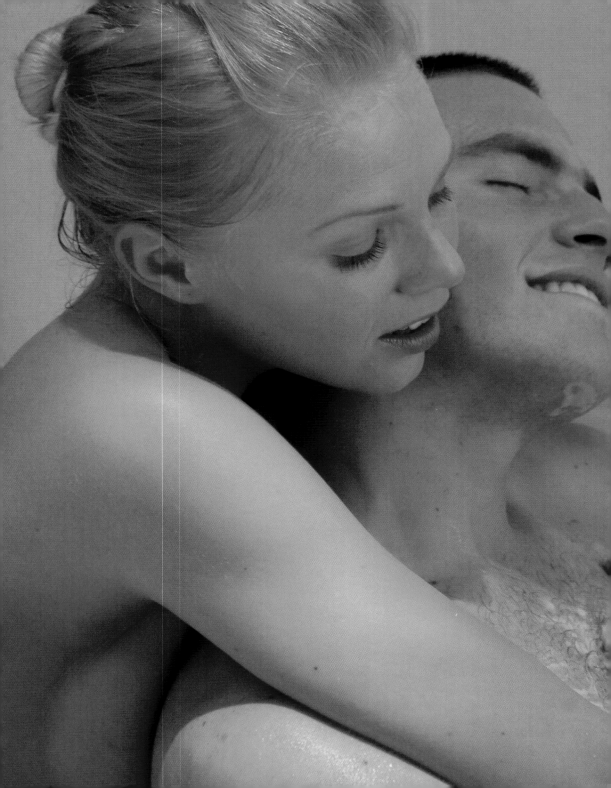

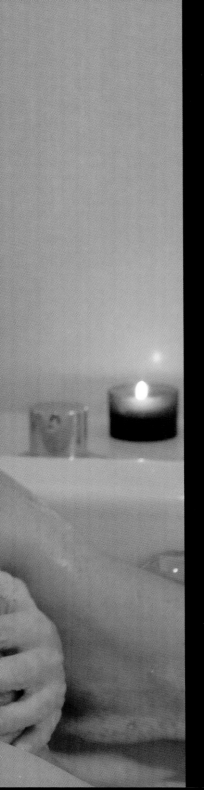

CHAPTER 3

Pre-sex secrets

If you're impatient to practice your lovemaking skills, I would urge you to wait a little longer. For impatience, anxiety, and even anger can form a crucial part in the build-up of sexual excitement. This may be explained by the arrangement of brain cells – those processing anger and anxiety are right next to those concerned with sexual excitement. The next chapter focuses on all the miraculous moves you can make as a prolonged prelude to intercourse.

Bedroom appeal

If you want to make a bedroom especially appealing to a man, it's worth remembering that he can get sexually excited solely by what he's viewing. There are certain decors, lights, wall hangings, and mirror reflections that put ideas into his head. The secret is to think about the atmosphere that will appeal especially to him. Is he a bondage man or is he an innocent? Will he adore a gothic atmosphere or would he be intimidated by anything other than pastels and florals? In your perfectly sexy bedroom he'll feel totally and individually spoiled by sensuality.

FEMININE BEDROOM

It's neat and it's tidy. The bed is made with clean, neutral sheets, the bedroom colors match and the curtains meet precisely in the middle. White muslin hangs over the bedstead lending a slightly tropical flavor to the environment. A candelabra is lit in advance of the man's arrival and the room is carefully pre-warmed. Clothes and cosmetics have been cleared carefully away and the crisp bed sheet is turned back enticingly.

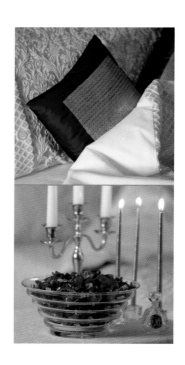

THE IMPRESSION IT MAKES ON A MAN

The male who lies back in this perfectly laundered and co-ordinated setting is going to feel very different to the guy who has to brush aside a pile of old socks and last night's pizza carton. The bedroom's owner is matter-of-fact with traditional values, but this room may become a surprise arena for wild sex.

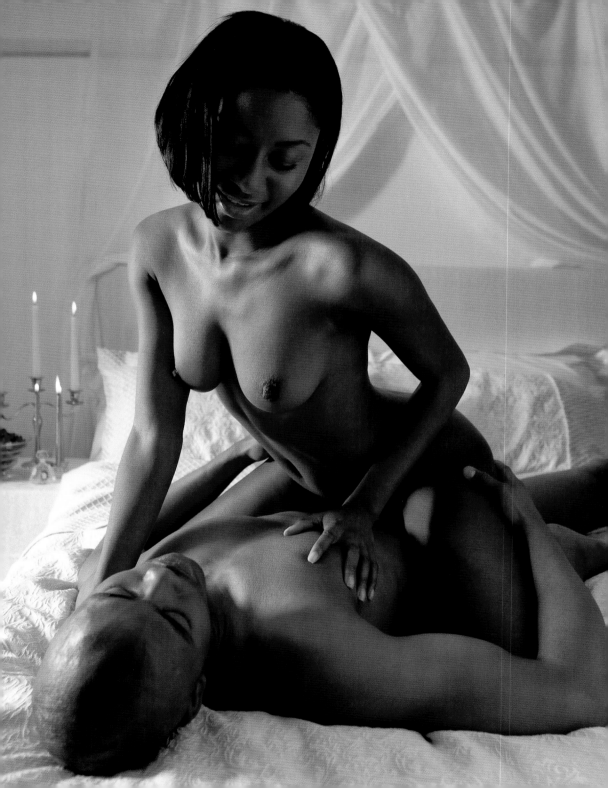

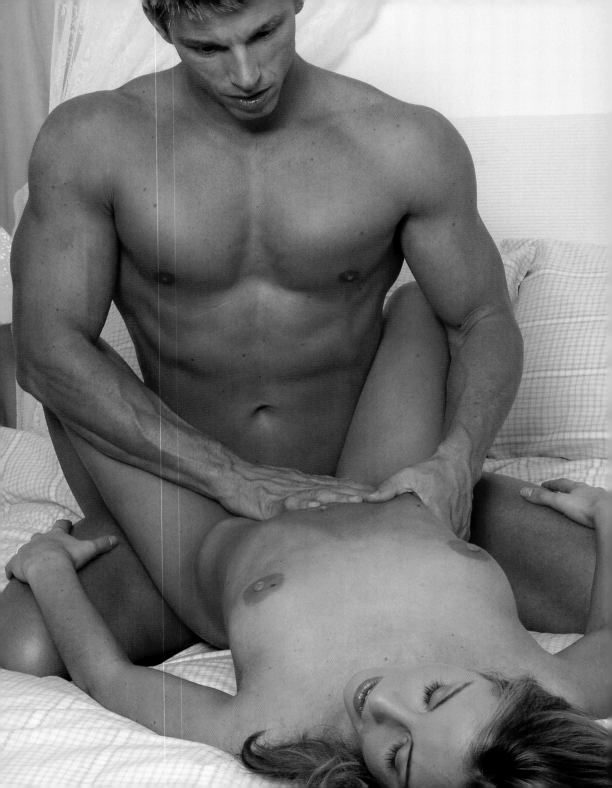

ROMANTIC BEDROOM

The four-poster bed is draped with white muslin in a feminine fashion and spread across the pure cotton sheets are beautiful pink rose petals. The bedroom's owner has ensured that the room smells heavenly — probably of rose perfume. There's one bedside lamp that throws out a pool of light, and arranged close to the bed is a full-length mirror that poses as a jewelry stand but just happens to reflect the bed's occupants.

THE **IMPRESSION** IT **MAKES** ON A **MAN**

The bedroom's owner has romantic ideas about sex and has probably read the *Kama Sutra*. This indicates that she is sexually knowledgeable but not necessarily widely experienced. The sheer femininity of the room might mean that she is longing to find out more and looks forward to sharing your enthusiasms.

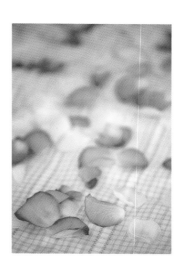

"Time-out" bedroom

At the other end of the spectrum, this secret area is an adjunct to a dark candle-lit bedroom. A door leads to a walk-in wardrobe, painted pitch black and with only a tiny violet light in a corner. As your man's eyes adjust he sees leather straps and chains attached to the wall and, hanging in neat rows, dog collars with spikes, a set of black whips, a pair of nipple clamps dangling, and a variety of toys used for domination and restraint. The door into the wardrobe has a large peephole from which you can either look in or out. Should you choose to look out — at the main bedroom — you see that the bed is directly in line with the peephole. Your man either runs like hell or rejoices that he's finally found someone who likes the same kind of games that he does.

❝ THE MORE DARING YOUR BEDROOM, THE MORE CERTAIN YOU SHOULD BE OF YOUR LOVER'S SEXUAL INCLINATIONS. ❞ *Anne*

SUMPTUOUS BEDROOM

The old-fashioned bedstead has bars at the head and is spread with striking red sheets, draped with scarlet ribbon and gold organza. On the side table is a pair of red furry hand cuffs. There's an old-fashioned drying rack at the side of the room from which hangs decorative scarves, artificial flowers, long bead necklaces, and one black-handled whip with long, brilliant latex flails.

Lighting is from a red lightbulb or shade with a couple of candles strategically placed nearby. On the dressing table is an array of brilliant jewel-colored vibrators, standing upright like an erotic rainbow. Placed in front of these are delicate pots of multicolored lubricants, and over the gold Victorian oval mirror hangs a black satin blindfold.

THE IMPRESSION IT MAKES ON A MAN

The room manages to be both mysterious and direct, which is rare. It feels immediately erotic and is full of objects that suggest bizarre but beautiful sexual practices. This elaborate setting indicates that the room's owner really knows what she's doing. The man, therefore, can expect a fantasy-like experience, perhaps in spite of her rather straight-laced appearance.

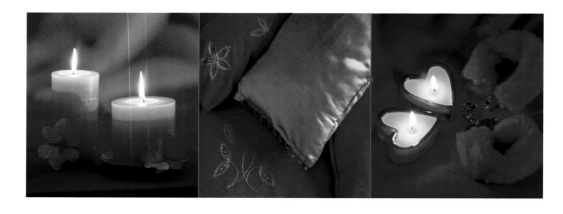

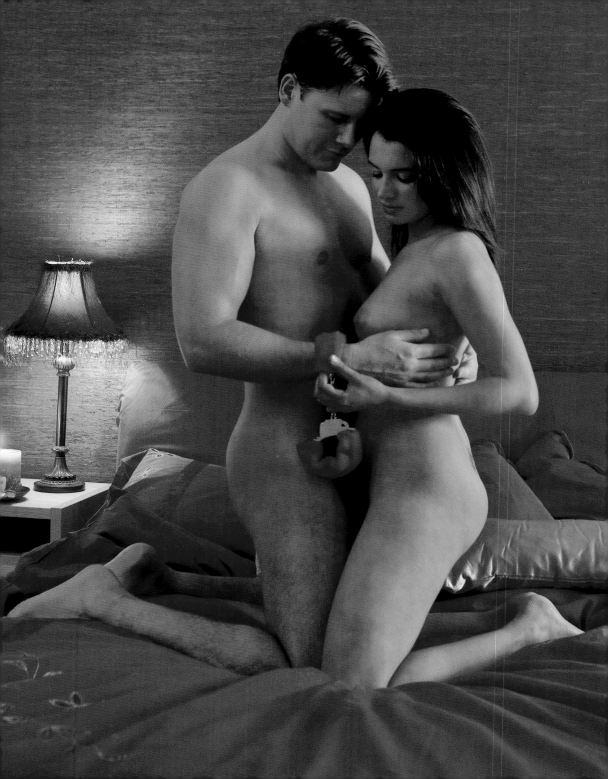

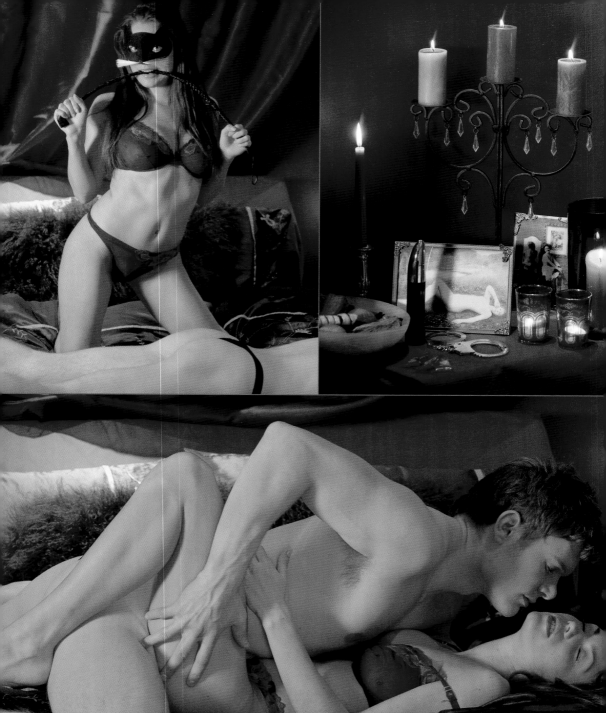

EROTIC BEDROOM

The bed is king-sized with dark silky sheets, and the door of the adjoining bathroom is open just far enough to show gleaming black tiles on the wall. At the foot of the bed is a huge chest, thrown open and containing material shot with silk and an array of black and white canes, whips, flails, cords, and blindfolds spilling over the sides. A black mask is dominant in this collection, along with several vibrators of different sizes on the bedside table. Lighting is from candles only, but it's sufficient to illuminate the art on the walls.

Powerfully erotic wall hangings and paintings are strong features in this intriguing room. They consist of *Leda and the Swan* and of Victorian and Edwardian erotic paintings of scantily clad women holding pitchers at angles that best show off their breasts.

THE IMPRESSION IT MAKES ON A MAN

When he looks at the wall hangings he immediately sees sex. The woman who lives in this type of bedroom is totally unashamed when it comes to lovemaking and is upfront about most aspects of it. The tasteful litter of sex toys falling out of the toy chest bears witness to this. A man can expect a very sexually knowledgeable person indeed in this environment. Some men, however, might find this room scary. There may be anxiety lurking in the back of the male mind about the kind of performance that this room warrants — be warned.

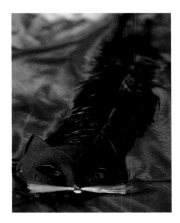

Impressions of sensuality

When preparing for exquisite sex, sensual props, such as fabrics and lighting, should be high on your list for consideration. Here are my eight favorite ways to heighten an erotic atmosphere.

AROUSING AMBIENCE

- **Invest in soft throws** Buy fake fur, a sheepskin rug, imitation tiger skins or a soft zebra bed quilt – anything that is sensual to the touch and looks exotic. Don't make the room too "pink and fluffy" because men don't find that kind of coziness sexy. Lend an erotic element to your furnishings because you want him to be a little on edge. You want him to feel sensual but not entirely comfortable – if he's slightly nervous he'll also be more easily aroused.

- **Smell sophisticated** A bedroom smelling of last night's fish supper is not sexy. Your room needs to be aired and cleaned regularly. If you're a smoker, don't stir without lighting a smoker's candle to mop up the stink of tobacco and always empty ashtrays and waste receptacles. Invest in a good-quality room spray. Avoid cheap ones at all costs or your room will just smell like a tart's boudoir. You want him to walk into your territory, sniff the scent of a beautiful woman, and experience prickles of anticipation down the back of his neck.

- **Sounding off** What kind of music sounds sensual to you? Are you someone who melts to Ella Fitzgerald or swoons to Norah Jones? Are you a passionate Rachmaninov aficionado or does Leonard Cohen make you seriously misbehave in intimate male company? Use melodies to nurture the erotic atmosphere, but don't overdo it.

> " THE LEAD-UP TO SEXUAL INTERCOURSE IS AS IMPORTANT AS THE ACT ITSELF. " *Anne*

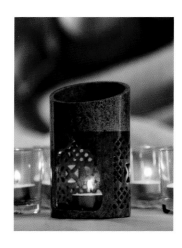

- **Low lighting** If you can't physically dim the lights, invest in lamps that throw out pools of light. Very bright lighting makes people feel vulnerable – in a negative way – whereas red or pink lightbulbs are incredibly flattering and sexy. You could break out the candles, but the drawback is that lighting them is a deliberate act. If you are planning a seduction, the fact that they are already alight appears arrogantly preplanned. Candles are perhaps best left for subsequent encounters.

- **Brain food** There are several ways to get pictorial ideas working erotically. A sexy statuette standing in a corner of the room is one, and an easel displaying an erotic painting is another. Explore the Internet for erotic art that suits your taste and consider having one or more prints framed.

- **Mirroring technique** Catherine the Great of Russia used to have the ceiling above her four-poster bed plastered with mirrors so that she could get a bird's eye view of her lovemaking. For those uneasy at the thought of such a great weight suspended above you, a full-length mirror on a stand at the side of the bed does almost as well.

- **The bed** Is it big enough? If you've ever tried making love on a small single divan you'll understand why I ask. The bed needs to be big enough to roll around on without falling off. It doesn't have to be king size but grown-up people need grown-up space.

- **The accessories** Positioned within arm's reach, but preferably not so that they are unavoidably obvious, you need such items as condoms, paper tissues, lubricant, vibrators, and any other sex toys you enjoy. If reading in bed is your thing, a small stack of sexy magazines or books is also in order.

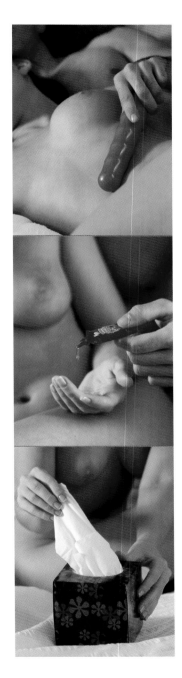

Sexy sound bites

A most disconcerting lover is the person who is completely silent in bed. You don't know if they're dumbstruck with joy or silently depressed. You've no idea if they like what you're doing since they give no feedback and your own ardor feels decidedly wobbly because of their apparent lack of pleasure. If this unresponsiveness applies to your lover, or to you, try my suggestions for expanding your sound bites.

TELL HIM ABOUT IT

- **Make some noise** It's not very difficult to make inarticulate sounds — to breathe heavily when you get turned on or to moan. Don't be afraid of sounding primitive — it's a great compliment to your lover.
- **Kiss him** If you feel passionate, show him by kissing him in a shower of tiny mouth movements. If you feel really passionate, bite him — not hard enough to hurt but hard enough to give him a pleasurable shock.
- **Shower him with praise** If your lover arouses you incredibly, tell him about it.

NOTHING TO SHOUT ABOUT?

If your lover's nothing to shout out about, maybe you shouldn't be with him. If he means well but isn't a very skillful lover, there are ways of asking him to change his technique without causing trauma. The best way to get a man to hone his love moves is assertion tempered by praise. You could say, for example, "I adore the way you stroke my breasts. If you could do the same thing to my clitoris that would be just amazing."

Therapy check UK sex therapist, Phillip Hodson, describes men as "praise-seeking missiles" and believes that you can never give a man too much! I would qualify this by saying you need to believe in what you're saying, at least at the time, otherwise there's a danger of sounding trite.

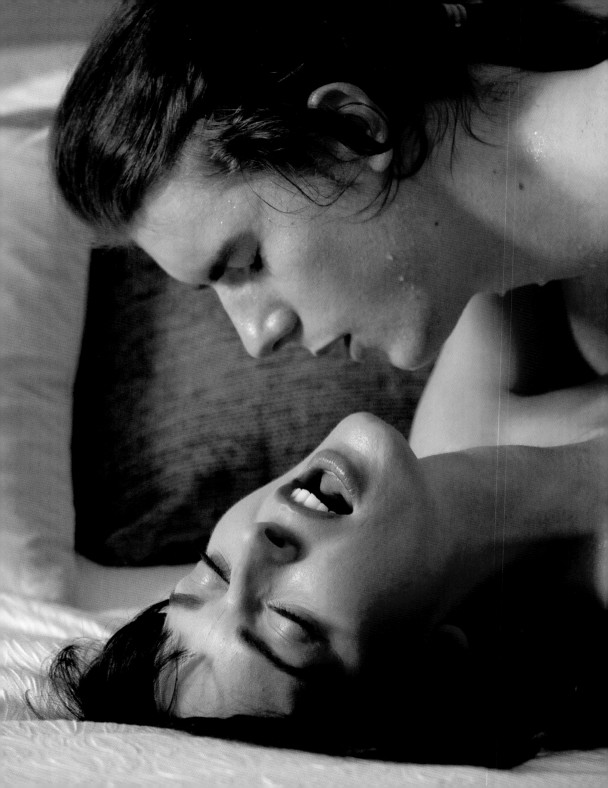

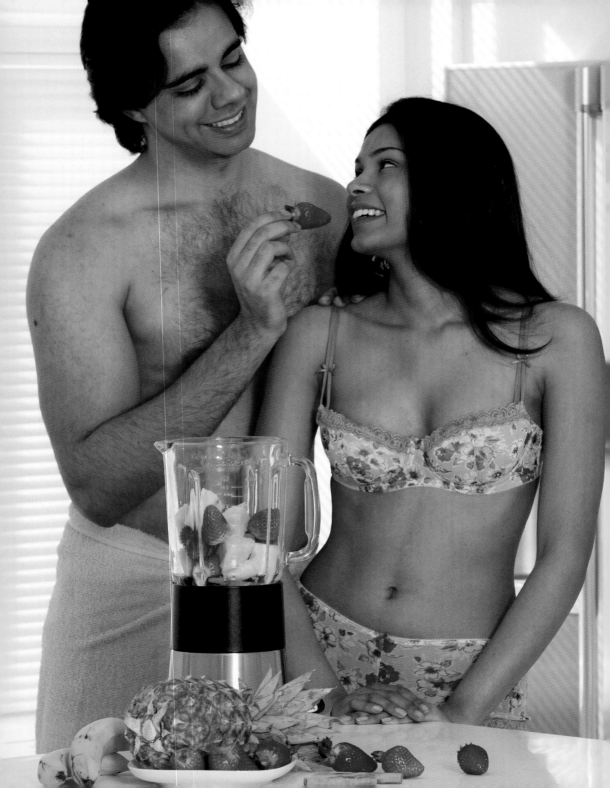

Spice up your juices

Each one of us possesses a very individual scent, which helps us to distinguish one another. To an extent we smell of what we eat as our perspiration "floats out" the essences of what we have recently ingested — especially on a hot day! Just as our perspiration reflects what we've been eating, so too do our vaginal juices and seminal fluid.

SWEET ENOUGH TO EAT

One of the problems many women have with giving oral sex is that the male ejaculate smells strong. The same is true for some men wanting to give oral sex to their female lover. However clean she may be, if her vaginal fluid smells of old broccoli, it's an ordeal rather than a delight. The secret to smelling sweet enough for oral sex depends on eating the right foods. It's commonly agreed that smoking makes bodily juices taste unpleasant and that if you cut down on salt, semen tastes sweeter. Interestingly, after eating red meat, semen will be thicker or gummier, according to Lou Paget (see p.219).

Sex secrets Xaviera Hollander suggests eating strawberries to combat bodily bitterness, while Lou Paget opts for fruit: "Melon, kiwi, or pineapples give you a lighter, sweeter taste," she says.

THE LOVE SMOOTHIE

Feed one another a sexy shake before lovemaking to make yourselves taste spicy. Blend together a banana, some strawberries, and pineapple with honey and, for a dash of the exotic, add nutmeg and cinnamon in tiny doses, being careful not to add too much spice.

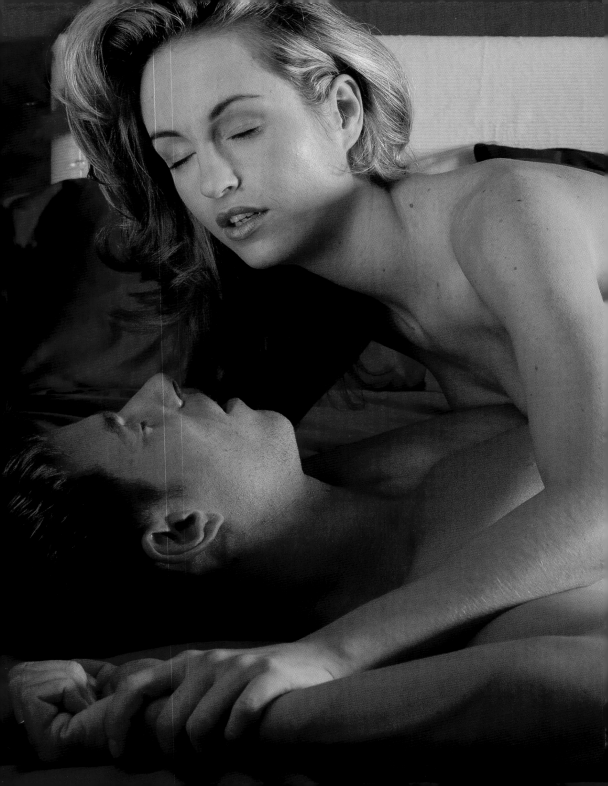

Unsexy intake

We all know that to a nonsmoking partner smoking is a potent lust-killer, but did you also know that in the long term tobacco impairs fertility and contributes toward male impotence? On the bright side, if you give up cigarettes by the age of 30 you can regain your health and live out your lifespan normally. Even if you give up later on you can still recover most of your good health.

THE **NOXIOUS WEED**

Recent health statistics on smoking also include marijuana. The weed, it seems, has an even higher tar content than ordinary tobacco making it bad for you for this reason alone, quite apart from the lethargy, depression, and more serious mental health problems that regular cannabis smoking can induce. The tar intake from marijuana smoking is greater in the absence of cigarette filters. The more heavily addicted you are to the stuff, the less sexy you feel. Cannabis addiction is at the root of many of the sexual-desire problems that come up in sex therapy clinics.

ONE TOO **MANY**

Alcohol is the other commonly used drug that seriously harms your sex life. Although it's true that a drink or two can loosen inhibitions when sexy feelings might be otherwise repressed, the minute you go beyond the first couple of glasses, your sex drive is impaired. This is because alcohol lowers the body's testosterone levels and testosterone is the body's sex fuel. Without it both sexes lose desire and erections refuse to show up when they're wanted.

Anne's advice Some prescription drugs adversely affect your sex life. These include: certain antidepressants (tricyclics, beta-blockers, and prozac); barbiturates and some other sleep-inducing drugs; some antihistamines and ulcer healing preparations; and many of the antianxiety drugs, such as propranolol. The major opiates deaden sensation generally and all types of tranquilizers impair sexual response. But the good news is that libido and sexual function usually reappear when the drugs are withdrawn.

Male pampering

People sometimes go for years without having another human being touch them. I refused to let my mother in the bathroom from the age of seven onward, I didn't have a boyfriend until I was 16, and I received my first massage aged 30. I remember the delight when someone finally focussed massage touch on me. Even though I was in a loving sexual relationship I was touch starved and missing out on a world of sensation.

THE **POWER** OF **PAMPERING**

I suspect men are much more starved for touch than women, which means that an occasional pampering session feels heavenly to them. A longing for touch or pampering may be one of the main reasons men pay for sex — they urgently need physical attention. Many men possess the fantasy of possessing a body slave to minister to their every sensual need, however taboo this may seem.

In a sensual bathing ritual (see pp.64–65), soap-sodden, slippery hands and fingers arouse physical sensations all over the skin and this can create a strangely mixed sense of eroticism. As the bathing massage is so gradual and carried out under the guise of "soaping," it may enable your lover to accept intimate moves that he wouldn't normally feel comfortable with. But reserve male pampering for special occasions or he may end up taking it for granted!

Fact check Several distinguishable spots on the male and female body have been observed in trials to trigger very specific sexual arousal. The areas identified are the G-spot in the vagina and the P-spot in the male anus — regions of the body that have tended to remain taboo.

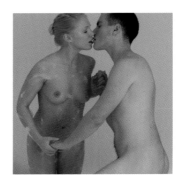

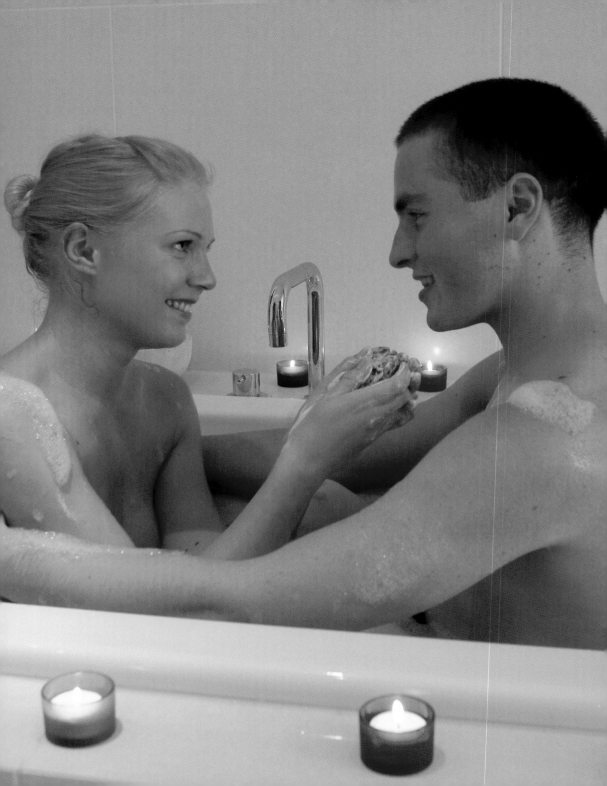

PAMPERING ROUTINE

- **Settle him** into the bath and, using a very sudsy gel or soap, slowly and sensuously wash him all over.
- **Let your fingers slip** into his most secret places as if by accident. You're ensuring that his testicles, perineum (area behind the testicles), and his anus are extra clean.
- **You might let** your soapy finger probe and massage his anus on the premise that it needs a lot of washing. If he's relaxed about it, push your finger in as high as possible.
- **Use your other hand** to simultaneously massage his penis with slow soapy strokes.

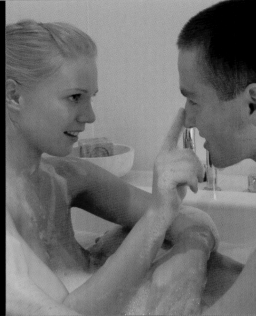

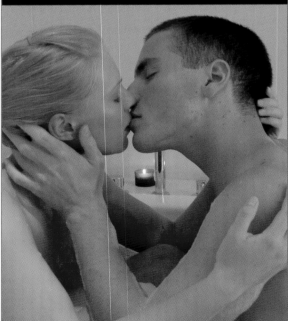

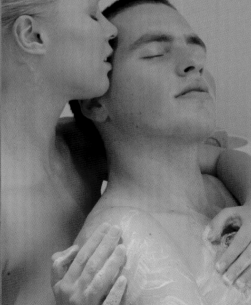

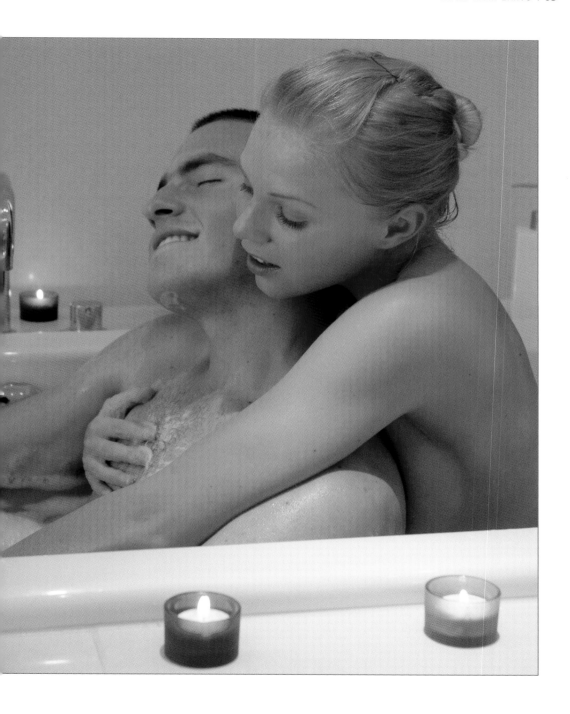

Sex stamina

If you want your partner to generate more sexual power and sex drive, try telling him about the US aerobic exercise specialists who noted that mice developed larger, firmer testes when they ran regularly on a treadmill. If your man's interested in enlarging this part of his anatomy, he could try regular running sessions, which will add to his general fitness as well. They will firm up the muscles at the top of his thighs at any rate, including those servicing his testicles, and firmer muscles in the genital area mean greater control over both testicles and penis.

TESTES TONING

US sex researchers Hartman and Fithian (see p.218), who have trained men to experience multiple orgasms, teach muscle control of the testes. They include this in their training programs because, by learning how to draw up the testes at will, many men are able to prevent ejaculation while still experiencing pleasure. In theory, they can then go on to enjoy further orgasms. In practice, most men find the further orgasms difficult to manage but, at the very least, testes toning means they can go on for much longer during intercourse and so prolong their general pleasure.

" STRONGER MUSCLES MEAN A STRONGER ORGASMIC RESPONSE BECAUSE HE'LL FEEL THE GENITAL CONTRACTIONS VERY POWERFULLY. " *Anne*

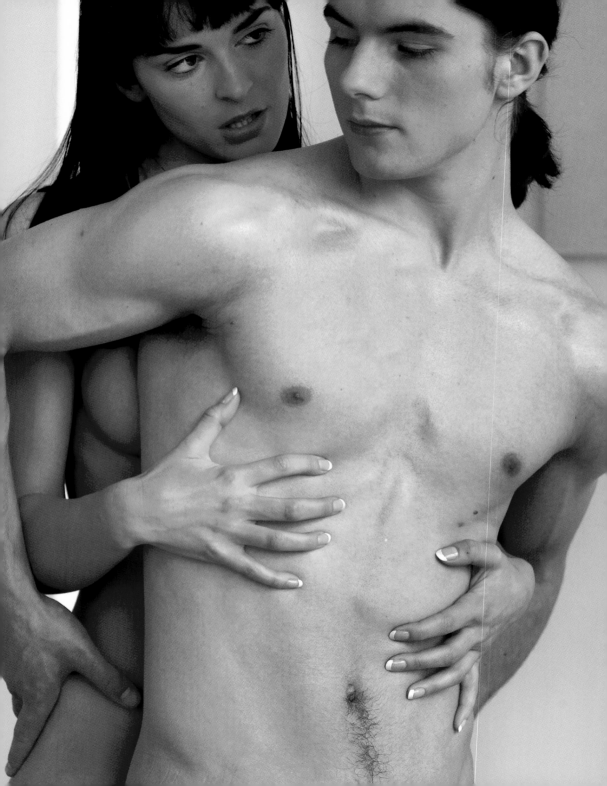

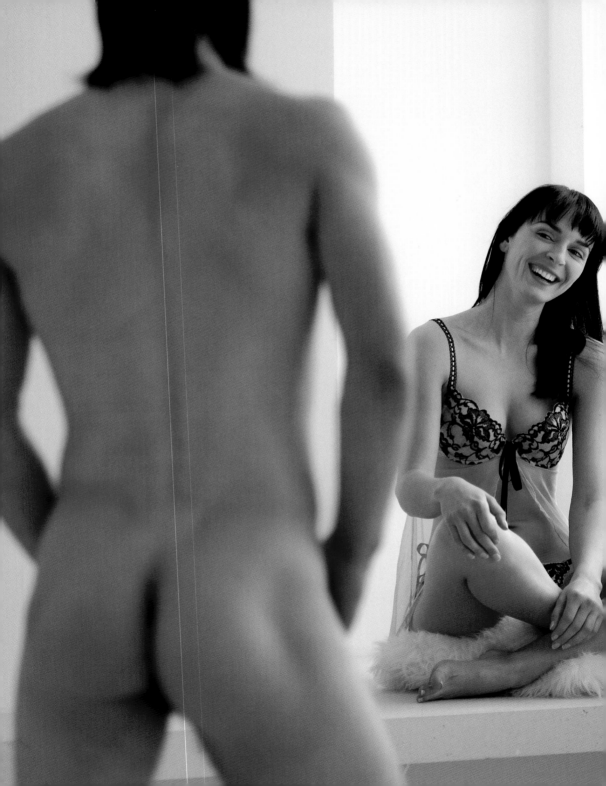

SEXUAL FITNESS – **FOR HIM**

Penis fitness may not be a phrase overheard too often in the gym and yet the penis is like any other part of the body in that it needs exercise. It gets exercised during masturbation, sex, and even urination, but there are also muscle "flexercises" for the genitals that actually improve the quality of male orgasms.

MALE MUSCLE **POWER**

A prerequisite for multiple orgasms is penis fitness because the ejaculate needs to be blocked, and this takes incredible muscle power. If a man can tense-and-relax his penis strongly enough, he can close off his penile channel at will, but serious training is required, as follows:

1 He "twitches" the penis ten times a session for at least three sessions a day.

2 "Raising the flag": he imagines that his penis has a flag on the end of it, which he has to pull up by degrees. He raises it about one third of the way, waits, then raises it halfway. He waits again, then raises it to the very top of the flagpole and holds it there for a count of five before lowering it again in gradual stages.

3 He should try these exercises on his upper thigh muscles, his buttock muscles, and on his anus to see if he can tell the differences in strength.

4 Next time he think he's going to climax, he could try to slow down, or even stop, his ejaculation. If he can do this – and it's very difficult – he is free to continue stimulation and try for another climax.

Anne's advice Once he can manage these exercises without difficulty his penile contractions will be stronger during orgasm so that climaxes will feel deeper and more powerful. The ultimate test of a truly fit penis is if you can hang a pair of lacy panties on it for five whole minutes.

Research check An underacknowledged event that can hamper your man's sex stamina is the male menopause, or andropause. Symptoms, including a lack of sexual potency, are due to falling levels of testosterone and they can be improved with testosterone replacement therapy. The average age of andropause onset is 50-plus, but like menopause, it can sometimes strike earlier.

SEXUAL FITNESS – **FOR YOU**

Flexing muscles may not be a priority for today's female self-improvers, yet some of the most legendary courtesans have flexed one particular set of muscles with profound success. Perhaps you've heard of the women who possess such supreme control of their vaginal muscles that they are able to massage a man from within? There are apocryphal tales of nightclub performers who can smoke a cigarette with a muscular vagina, and instructions by Tao writers direct women to pleasure their men using vaginal contractions alone. The man literally doesn't move but is stimulated to orgasm nonetheless.

VAGINAL AEROBICS

1 Practice squeezing the vagina tight as if you were attempting to stop the flow of urine midstream. Then let go. If it helps, practice squeezing on a pencil or a finger (if you can't feel it, you need to try harder). Do this squeeze-relax sequence ten times a session and try to do at least six sessions a day.

2 After a week of practicing the first exercise, try "fluttering." This means doing the squeeze-relax exercise in quick succession. Do this six times a day. The objective is to extend the length of time you can sustain the fluttering.

3 A week later, add the "hydraulic elevator" to your repertoire. Imagine the interior of your vagina as an elevator shaft. Squeeze your vagina closed in order to get the elevator up a floor. Hold the elevator there for a short time before squeezing tighter and taking the elevator up to the next floor. Hold the elevator again for a short time and then go right on up to the top floor. Hold it there, then descend again, stopping at the next floor down and only relaxing when you arrive on the bottom floor again.

Anne's advice There are two reasons why you might want to privately practice vaginal aerobics. The first is that a toned up vagina experiences orgasm as a much stronger sensation, and the second is that you can grip your lover's penis while he's inside you – and he'll like that!

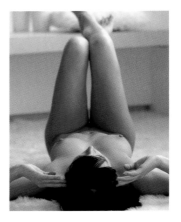

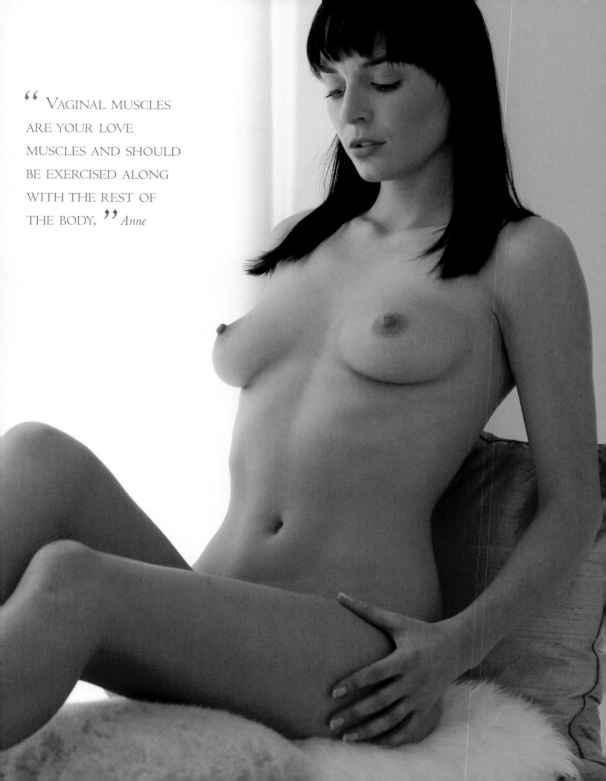

" VAGINAL MUSCLES
ARE YOUR LOVE
MUSCLES AND SHOULD
BE EXERCISED ALONG
WITH THE REST OF
THE BODY. " *Anne*

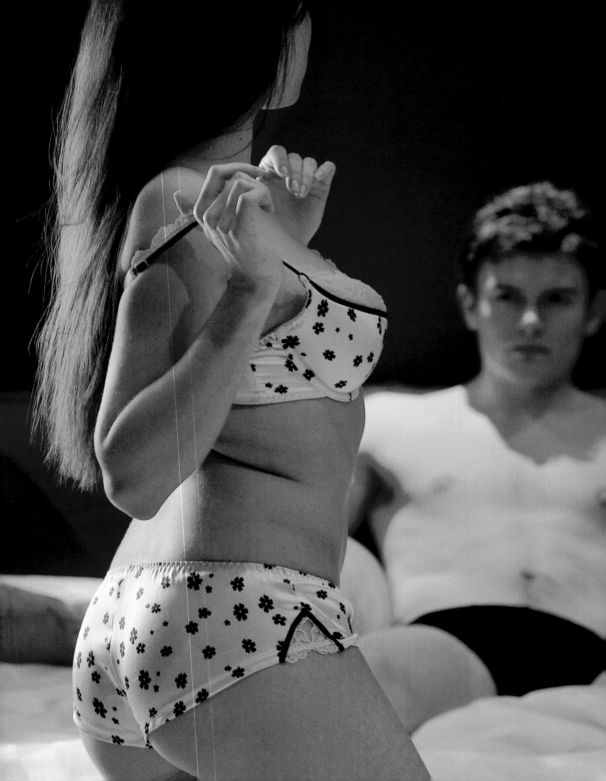

CHAPTER 4

Linge
loving

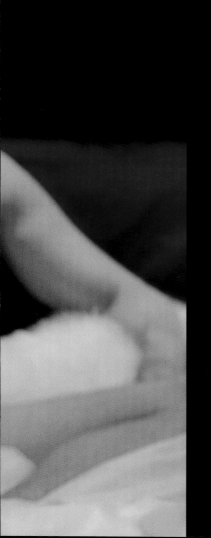

One of the grea
make is to rush
women do this
they're impatien
not sure what e
desperate for se
becomes routine
particularly wor
following chapt
timeless secrets
There are nume
to linger over se
need extra time,
almost childlike

Wait-for-it games

Like most good things, truly erotic sex is something to be lingered over, taken slowly and deliberately, and thought about a great deal. If you're just getting to know someone, spinning out your time together without having intercourse can result in a very sexy buildup of excitement. If you're already lovers, postponing sex for a while can make the relationship feel like a new one again. The secret is to play "wait-for-it" games without letting your lover know what you're doing.

WHY THESE WORK

Wait-for-it games are based on a tantric-style approach to prolonging and enriching intercourse known as *karezza*. The term was coined in the US during the 19th century by Dr. Alice Bunker Stockham for her classifications of nonreligious sex practices. Wait-for-it games operate on both physical and emotional levels. On the physical side, the buildup of sexual tension (resulting in muscular contractions in the sex organs) means that, on eventual release, the resulting orgasm is longer and stronger than it might be if you enjoyed one nightly.

I don't advise you to try this all the time, however. Weighed up against "waiting for it" is the fact that you're missing out on many precious climaxes, even if they are less powerful!

CREATING EROTICISM

On the emotional side, you're building up the idea of sexuality in your brain. Because you can't have sexual fulfillment, you're thinking about it more, and the longer you last with this waiting, the more tantalized you and your partner become.

Anne's advice Focus on the sensuality of all-over body excitement. You may be surprised to find that after wait-for-it games, the entire body is so eroticized that orgasm is only one small part of the incredible experience.

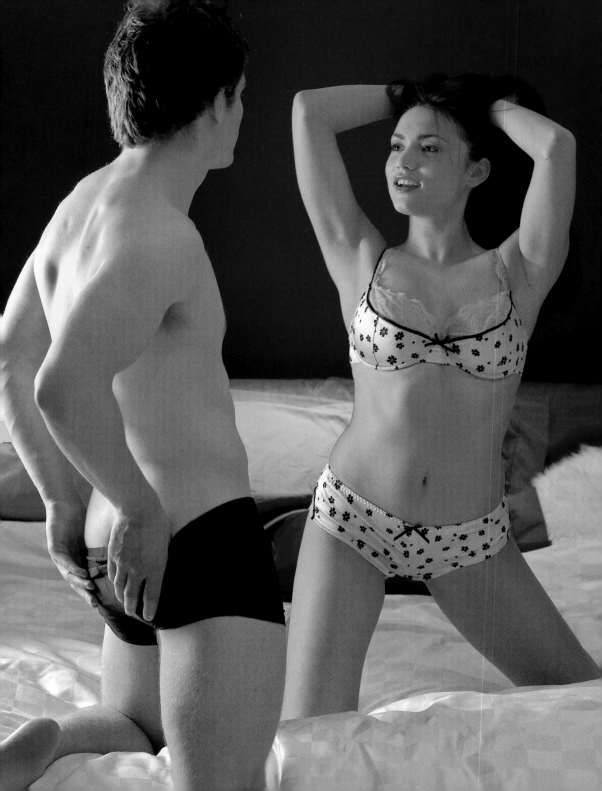

WITHHOLD FOR A WEEK

- **Make an agreement** between yourselves that however desperately you want orgasms you'll hold back for a week.
- **You're allowed** to make love in every possible way, but not to climax. Don't give in to the temptation to masturbate.
- **Stimulate each other** by hand…by tongue…and by rubbing your entire bodies against each other.
- **Don't be afraid** of nearing orgasm, but always stop when you recognize the warning signals.

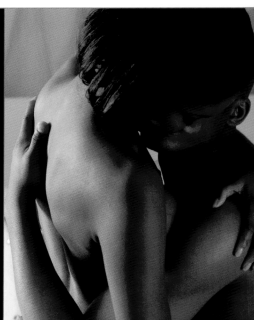

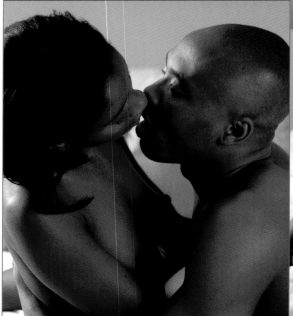

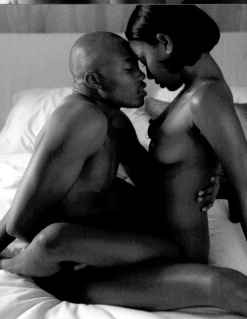

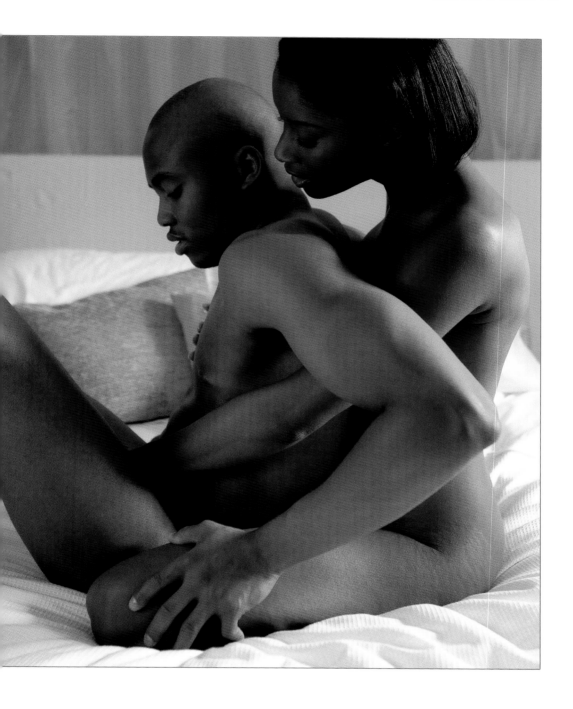

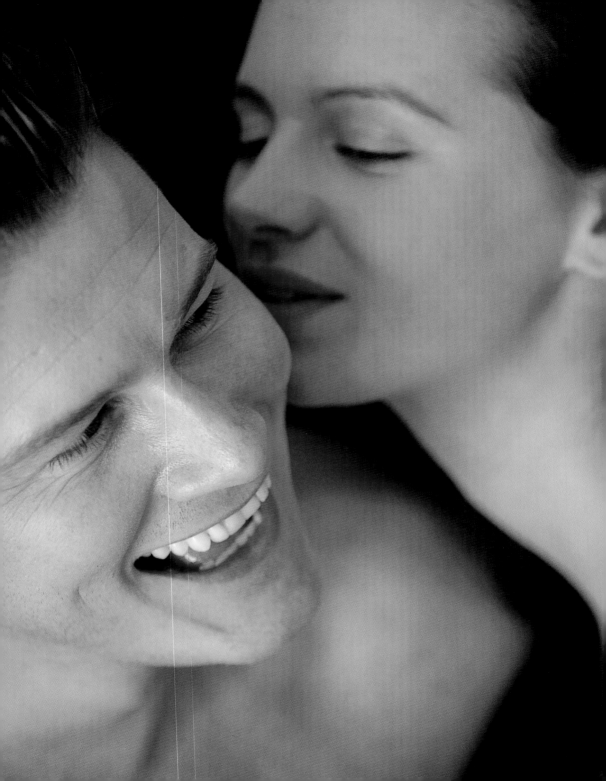

TEASE WITHOUT TOUCHING

The more something is promised to you and the longer you
are forced to wait for it, the greater the buildup of anticipation.
And anticipation is, in itself, sexually arousing. This routine for
increasing anticipation is one to take your time over. The secret
is to excite your man while showing no signs that you actually
intend to go further.

TEASING ROUTINE

- **Explore** all the sexy spots on your lover's body.
- **Lick** his navel and add a few tiny nips of the teeth, as if
  you're doing it by accident.
- **Work** on the area behind his knees. A cluster of light kisses
  here will set him all of a flutter...so too will the same moves
  on his shoulder blades.
- **Blow** kisses in his ears then lick and chew his earlobes.
- **Suck** his fingers one by one then his toes, then gently kiss
  across his buttocks and especially his scrotum.

WHY THIS WORKS

There are many powerfully sensual erogenous zones that are
either forgotten or never discovered. This routine enables you
to explore them. Each time you tease a sexy part of the body,
local nerve endings send messages to the brain saying, "this
feels amazing." The brain, in response, sends messages to
the penis saying, "this feels so good you might want to do
something about it." The result is one highly stimulated
penis without a stroke being laid upon it.

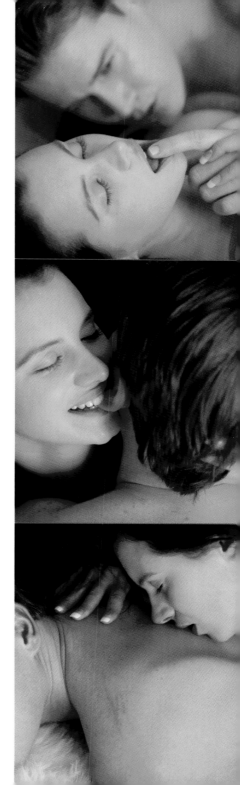

Changing pace

Your man is so attractive you long for your lovemaking to go on forever. It's a shock therefore to discover that he is so turned on by you that he's overwhelmed — with the result that he climaxes far too fast. You're just getting into your stride when he's already finished. The result is one very frustrated female. Fortunately, all many men need is to get used to your amazing presence and very soon their staying power will increase. Should he continue to climax too quickly, there are lots of ways to calm him.

SLOWING HIM DOWN

Sex educator Steve Bodansky (see p.218) claims that you usually only have to change the strokes that are stimulating your lover to slow down proceedings. So, if you're masturbating him by hand with a particular stroke, change the pressure and direction of stimulation. While you're having intercourse, alter the position. If you're on top, for example, roll over sideways and go for a side-by-side position. This position will be much less stimulating for him.

THE SQUEEZE TECHNIQUE

This is the method made famous by US sex researchers, Masters and Johnson in the late 1960s and early 1970s (see p.219). If your man is reaching "the point of no return," he should reach down with his hand and squeeze his penis hard on the coronal ridge between fingers and thumb (see right). This blocks the expulsion of ejaculate. Masters and Johnson taught this technique to females and you can use it too, as long as your lover indicates when he's reaching bursting point.

SQUEEZE TECHNIQUE

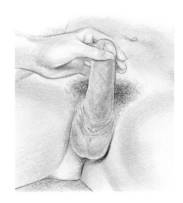

Squeeze the top of penis firmly between fingers and thumb.

You can quickly scoot down his body and apply the squeeze yourself. Then you massage his erection back into life so that intercourse can continue without interruption.

THE **BEAUTRAIS MANEUVER**

This changing-pace technique is named after the sex therapist, Pierre Beautrais, who documented it in New Zealand. It's one that the man must do for himself without your assistance. Again, as he approaches bursting point, he reaches behind his testicles and firmly pulls them down. This constricts ejaculation by blocking the urethral passage and allows you both to prolong your lovemaking.

THE **JEN-MO** POINT

This is a Taoist method of preventing ejaculation. Pressing hard on the perineum with an index or middle finger constricts the ejaculate. The Jen-Mo point is an acupressure point on the perineum, halfway between the anus and the scrotum (see right). Tao teachers warn, however, that you need to be accurate about which point you press. The dangers are that if you apply the pressure too close to the anus it won't work but if you press too close to the scrotum, the semen will go into the bladder making the urine cloudy.

DRUG TREATMENT

If nothing else works there are now prescribed drugs (most notably beta-blockers) that can delay your partner's orgasm. Beta-blockers are generally prescribed for angina, high blood pressure, and irregular heart rhythms and are a family of drugs that includes Propranolol. A side effect of these medications is that they reduce sexual desire and make climaxing more difficult, but they should only be used as a last resort for this purpose.

Sex secrets Pressing the Jen-Mo point can improve the quality of the male orgasm as well as prolong intercourse by preventing ejaculation. Semen is blocked from leaving the body and is reabsorbed in the blood. In Taoism and sexual Kung Fu, this point is called "point of a million gold coins."

JEN-MO POINT

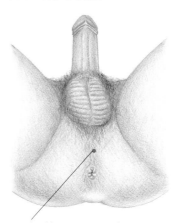

Jen-Mo acupressure point (halfway between testicles and anus)

Press the Jen-Mo point firmly using an index or middle finger.

SPEEDING HIM UP

It may not happen often, but sometimes your man is unable to climax. There he is, seriously turned on by your ministrations, but the action seems to go on and on. Although you're flattered by his continued interest, you're also getting tired. Or maybe he can't get as far as intercourse because he's finding it difficult to keep his erection. The reasons for this are varied and sometimes complicated, but here are some imaginative techniques that can speed up your man's arousal and seriously hasten his orgasm.

HANDS ON

When you're straddled above him in the woman-on-top position, reach down with one hand and, grasping his penis with the whole hand, use your hand as an extension of your vagina. Let it rise and fall as your body rises and falls so that his penis is receiving an extra long stimulation. Your hands also grip him much more tightly than your vagina can alone. If part of the problem is that his penis has lost some of its sensitivity then this approach can put you back on track.

THE FRENULUM

This is the bandlike ligament that links the ridge on the underside of the penis with the penis shaft (see also p.120). It's full of nerve endings and just titilating this part of the penis can make some guys super-responsive. Ring your hand around the ridge of the penis and lightly and quickly move your hand up and down focusing the touch on the frenulum. He'll respond to this well – it's a promise!

STROKE HIS P-SPOT

"P" stands for perineum in this context. This stretch of skin between the base of the penis and the anal opening is a well-kept sex professionals' secret. It's a hidden pleasure spot and the

Anne's advice The speed of the male sexual response changes with advancing age. During the "excitement phase" of sex, his erection may be delayed, making more direct stimulation of the penis necessary. And the erection may not be as firm as it was in his youth.

FRENULUM

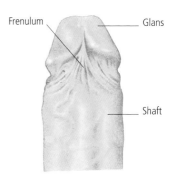

Frenulum — Glans

— Shaft

Licking or stroking this sensitive area will invariably speed things up.

best way to show your man its power is to press it with your fingers. This pressure sends waves of sensation throughout his genitals. Make the pressure firm, pressing down into the skin and move the pressure backward and forward or in a circle. You're not moving your fingers on his skin; you're actually rotating the tissue underneath his skin. If you want to practice in advance, try it out on your own perineum. You'll also find this a very pleasurable pressure zone.

RING ROUND THE MOON

This takes the stroking of the perineum a bit further. Make sure your forefinger is well lubricated, place it on the outside of his anal entrance and run it lightly clockwise, then counterclockwise, increasing the pressure as you go. The anal opening is rich in sensational nerve endings. (See also pp.136–141.)

Sex secrets Anyone believing that anal stimulation has to hurt is misguided. With its high concentration of nerve endings, the anus can be painful when mistreated, yet it can be a source of great pleasure. The secret is to go slowly and to give the anal muscles plenty of time to relax.

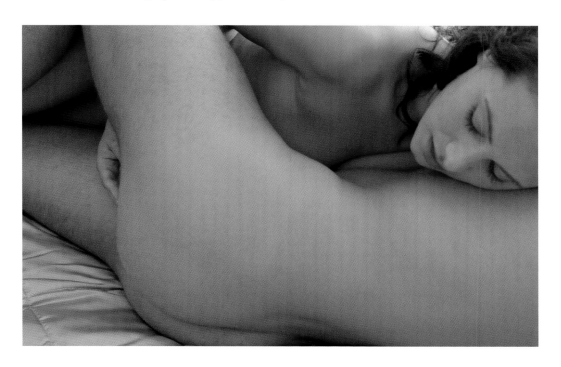

Sheer eroticism

The use of external stimuli is only one way to get sexually excited – eroticism can be heightened by spending time deliberately doing absolutely nothing. Erotic movie star, Annie Sprinkle (see p.219), advocates "nothing sessions" to sharpen up your sense of perception, and I've added a couple of other suggestions for experiencing eroticism without physical contact.

THE **"NOTHING"** SESSION

Set a timer for thirty minutes and lie in a quiet, private room, either clothed or unclothed. Lie facing your partner and look into each other's eyes. If you are not used to doing this you may feel uncomfortable but don't analyze your feelings – just allow yourself to enter a trancelike state and go with your feelings. When the timer sounds, end your reverie with a warm kiss then share your thoughts.

THE **EROTIC** PRESENT

Wrap up an object of curiosity in beautiful paper. You might offer a strangely shaped candle, a beautiful pink feather, or an old-fashioned erotic picture.

TELEPHONE SEX

Practiced by couples forced to spend time apart, telephone sex can feel surprisingly real. Tell your partner your hot feelings over the phone. Better still, stimulate yourself while telling him you imagine it's him who's making you aroused. Your arousal can be heard in your voice, which is very exciting for him.

Anne's advice An erotic present should be something out of the ordinary so that the recipient will have to use his imagination to work out what is meant by the gift.

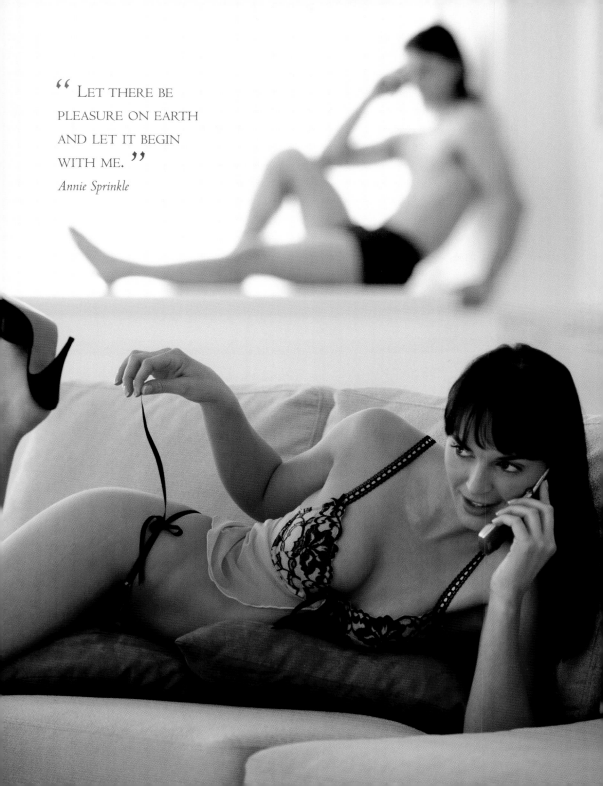

"Let there be
pleasure on earth
and let it begin
with me."
Annie Sprinkle

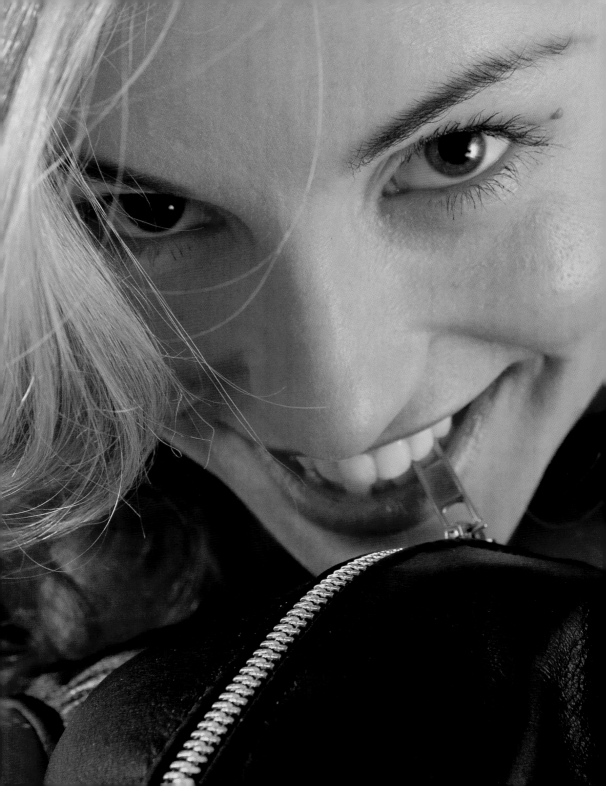

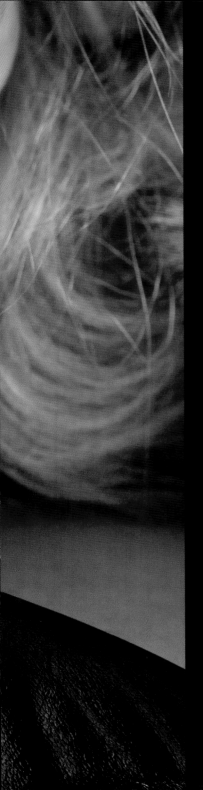

CHAPTER 5

Men's sexual fantasies

Fantasy is a powerful mental tool. Thousands of men and women secretly fantasize as a way of reaching and enhancing climax. Along with many other sex therapists, I believe that fantasy is an entirely natural part of a legitimate sex life. The mind plays an essential part in how both men and women experience desire, excitement, and orgasm. These pages provide a vivid insight into some of the most common male fantasies for you to consider working into your sex life.

Enter his imagination

The truth is that most men long for women to enter into their sexual imaginations and take part in them. Yet women don't always understand or appreciate this. Many women believe that men will think less of them if they develop a truly raunchy side to their character. But if you have a solid relationship with your lover, sharing sexual experiences and true erotic ambitions will inevitably deepen the bond between you.

THE **RISKS**

There may be other fears attached to confessing your greatest secret desires to each other. Perhaps you don't want to run the risk of spoiling your fantasies by exposing them to the light of day? And if you act out a fantasy together, isn't there a real chance that it might not turn you on again? Before taking action, it's sensible to take a hard look at reality. Yes, there are risks attached. Once you've acted out a fantasy a few times, there is the chance that it will lose its attractions. What you can control in you mind can't be controlled in reality, and some people do find that by revealing their secret, the fantasy loses its power.

THE **JOYS**

Anything new and exciting, however, involves risk. Taking a risk means giving yourselves the chance to move on to new and exciting ground. You may, for example, find that you have the most amazingly imaginative love life once you're able to open up about what really excites you both. Your relationship may grow deeper and far more meaningful because you've dared to say things you've never said before and you've had them accepted.

Research check Dr. Glenn Wilson, at the British Institute of Psychiatry, has made a remarkable scientific study of the sexual imagination. He states that fantasy is directly related to sexual libido. The greater your sex urge, the higher is your likelihood of having sexual fantasies.

THE **UNDECIDED**

Some of us are risk takers and some aren't. But there's also a bunch of men and women who fall in between such categories. We hesitate but we'd like to find out what lies on the "other side" of sex. If only we could find the courage, if only we knew the best ways to tackle such a challenging issue, we might try something new. The "in-betweens" can take some comfort from the following facts:

- If you lose a fantasy because you've revealed it, other fantasies will move in to take its place.
- Fantasies can develop and change but still retain their former intensity.

FROM **IMAGINATION** TO **REALITY**

1 Start by sharing one of your fantasies then ask your lover to reveal one of his in return.

2 Resolve to use both sets of fantasies by talking about them openly in bed – telling them like stories, and perhaps taking the critical step of acting them out. These steps can be taken in a gradual progression. The advantage of such a gentle approach is that you can stop at any stage if you feel uncomfortable or if it seems like things are going too far.

3 If you both want to seriously act out a fantasy, accept that it might not work. It's important to negotiate this in advance so that your relationship remains uncomplicated.

4 Remember to take things gradually and to keep communicating with each other.

Research check Dr. John Bancroft, head of the Kinsey Institute in Indianapolis, has found a link between high testosterone levels and a greater ability to fantasize. The higher levels of testosterone that men have compared with women are also thought to be responsible for greater sex drive.

" OUR IMAGINATIONS NATURALLY EQUIP US FOR ALL KINDS OF MIND-BLOWING SEX. " *Anne*

PICKING HIM UP IN A BAR

- **If picking up a hooker** in a bar is his fantasy, don't tell him in advance what you intend, just make a date to meet at a local bar.
- **Make sure you're there** well in advance and perch on a stool by the counter. Naturally you're wearing a low neckline and an extremely short skirt.
- **Then just pretend** you're picking him up. Let him know your fee and warn him that no kissing is allowed. And when you lead him off to your room (either a hotel room or one lent by a friend), you make the moves. Don't let him take charge – this is his treat.

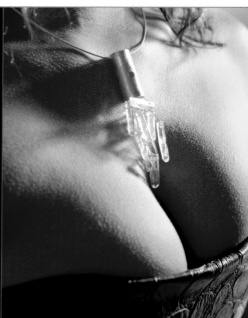

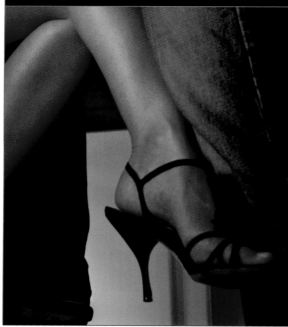

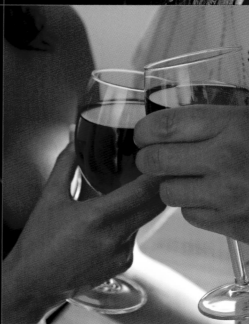

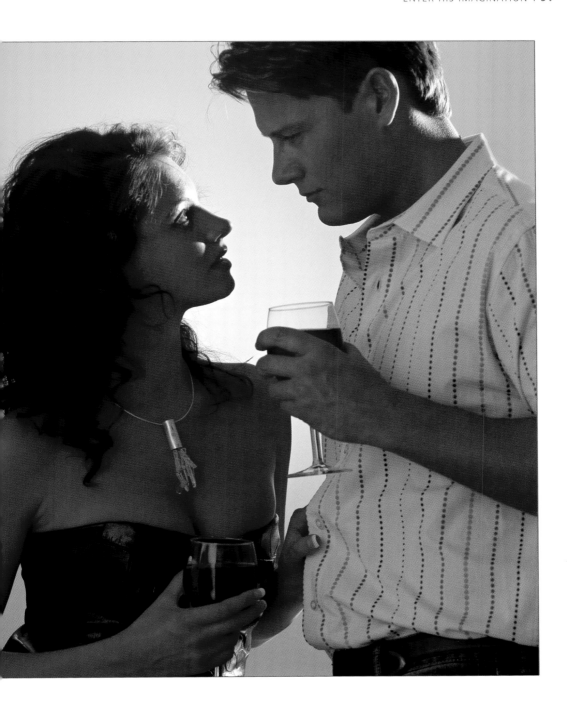

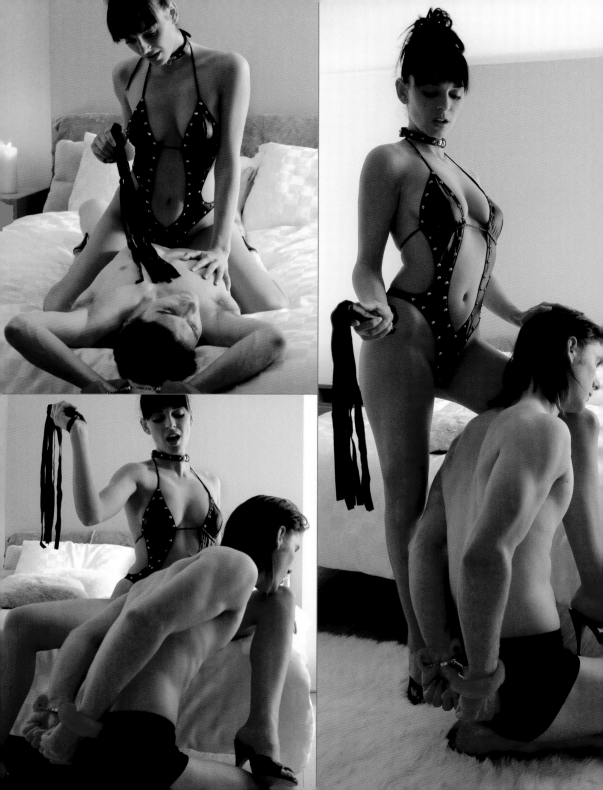

Going further

Punishment and bondage are among men's most common sex fantasies. If you know he's interested, try greeting him one day clad entirely in tight-fitting black leather or PVC. If you need inspiration, there are some amazing fashion companies manufacturing gorgeous rubber and leather outfits (see p.220). Experiment by keeping these clothes on when you have sex rather than taking them off!

PUNISHMENT **GAME**

Start off gently by taking all his clothes off. Explain that you are going to play a special game and agree on a password that he can use if he wants you to stop at any time. Tie a soft black blindfold or silk necktie around his eyes. Once he can no longer see, his other senses are enhanced and he feels vulnerable. Get him to kneel down and gently push his head forward until his forehead is touching the floor. This is a highly submissive pose and he will feel anxious anticipation. Pull his hands behind his back and tie them together. Point out to him that he is utterly in your power and that if he doesn't do exactly as you order, you will punish him.

ADD A LITTLE **HUMOR**

Punishment games aren't just about providing the recipient with pleasurable pain. Played cleverly, they can be humorous episodes, arranged in such a way that the recipient is unable to win, no matter what he does.

Anne's advice Work out what your partner wants to take in the way of punishment and incorporate it in the game. Don't impose your own ideas. If you're spanking him by hand, remove all rings and jewelry first, and if you're tempted to use a cane lightly, try the instrument out on your own hand first.

THE GRATITUDE GAME

- **Use a flat bendy paddle** whip or a latex flail to strike him across the buttocks, telling him he must say "thank you."
- **If he forgets**, because he's carried away with the eroticism of the stroke, he must be penalized with another stroke.
- **If he doesn't sound** enthusiastic enough, paddle him harder.
- **If he sounds too** enthusiastic, accuse him of overdoing it.
- **Make him count** the strokes while he's thanking you, but then insist he's got it wrong even if he hasn't.

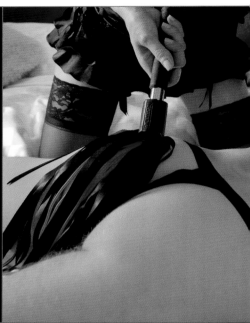

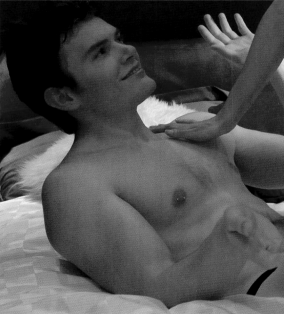

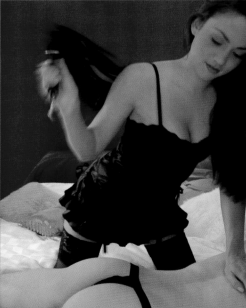

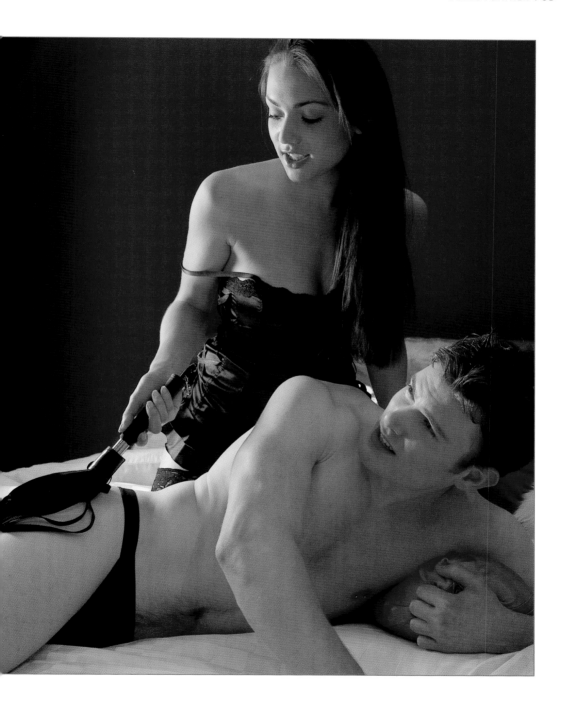

Going further still

Spanking and caning may sound like violent, painful activities but the appeal is that they accelerate desire. I am talking about sex games between lovers, not enemies. Should you need reassurance, consider the fact that a light slap on the buttocks brings the blood pleasantly to the surface. It may give you a shock — but the shock is exciting! Heat tingles and warms the skin and acts as a precursor to sexual excitement.

THE **FRUSTRATION** GAME

The secret of this game is to let your partner think you'll make one move, then when he's tensed and ready for it, make a different one. The frustration will arouse him and increase his sexual excitement. Give your man choices. You can start by offering him a choice between spanking by hand or with a paddle. Next you ask where he'd like it, indicating "here or there?" When he says "here" then spank somewhere else. And instead of using his choice of hand or paddle, use the opposite. When he protests spank him somewhere else again. From time to time you'll spank him in the requested place, but by this stage, it will confuse and excite him even more.

Anne's advice To spank without hurting use the flat of your hand not your fingers. Don't strike repeatedly in the same place and never spank on bony areas. Fleshy areas like the buttocks are the best. If your ministrations cause real pain you should stop. Agree on a codeword in advance that means the game should end.

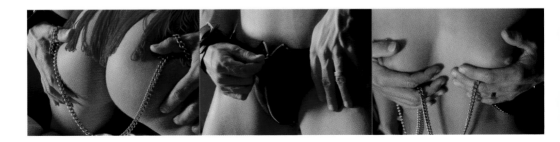

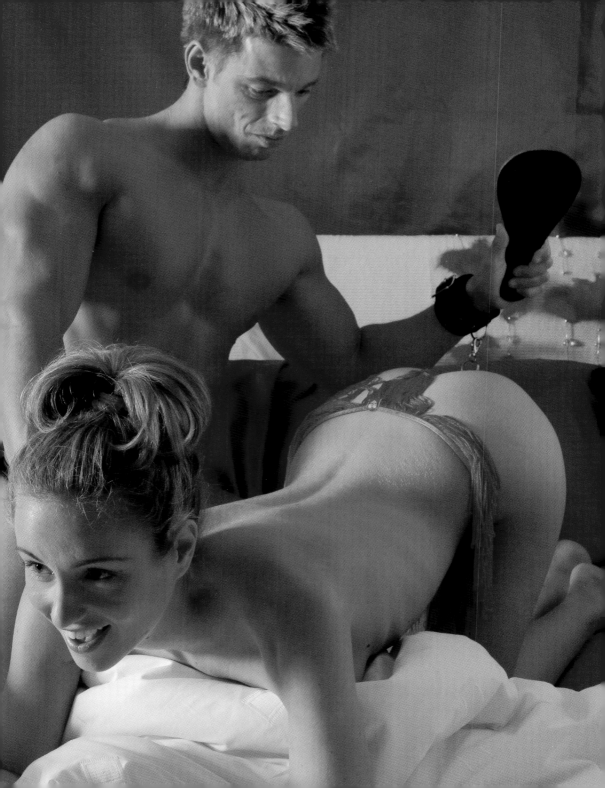

WRESTLING IN OIL

In this slippery sex game you and your lover are pretending to be all-in wrestlers.

- **Protect the floor** or choose a washable surface for your messy contest.
- **Strip yourself naked,** then strip him.
- **Next lubricate both** of you in liberal quantities of massage oil.

- **Tell him that the winner** of this wrestling match is the one who manages to stay on top of the other one for three minutes – obviously he will win and the prize is of his choosing.
- **An alternative is** to wear minimal clothing and the winner is the first one to take the other's underwear off.

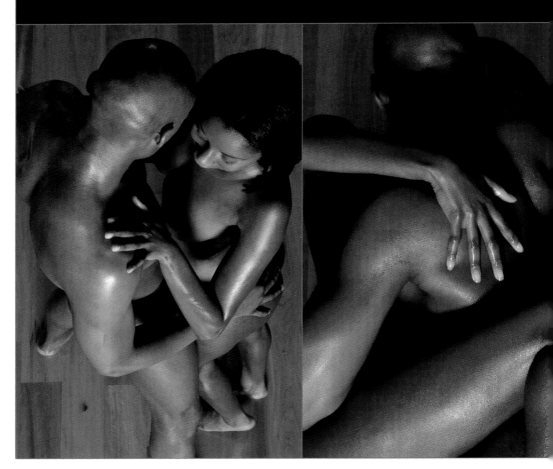

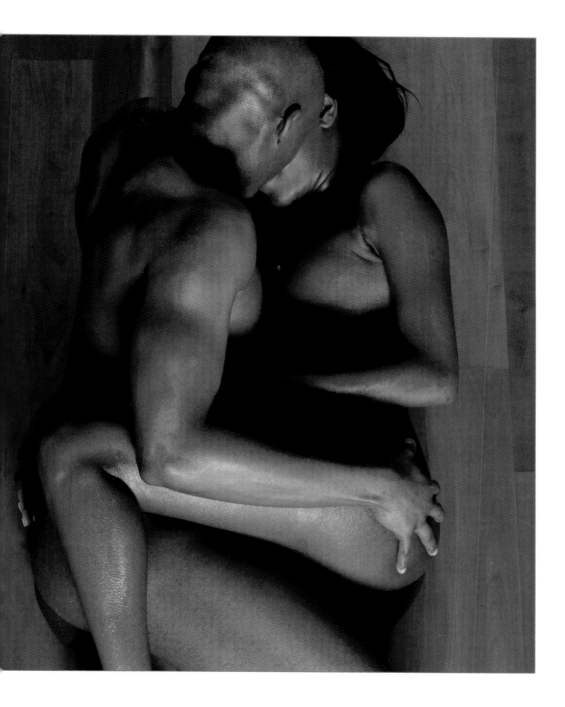

A stranger calls

This fantasy makes full use of the element of surprise, which is a powerful sexual turn on. There's a knock at the door and your lover opens it, expecting the plumber you told him you booked. Instead, he finds you waiting for him in an overall, with enough cleavage showing to hint at the stunning underwear you're wearing beneath the dirty work clothes.

THE **FANTASY UNFOLDS**

"You called for a plumber," you gently remind him. The studs on the front of your overall are extra-large, industrial size, and you toy with the top stud as you wait to be invited through. "I'm not surprised you've called me out," you say as you begin to step inside, "it's incredibly hot in here. Something must have gone wrong with your heating."

THE **TEMPERATURE** RISES

Unable to stand the soaring temperature a moment longer, you slowly begin to unfasten the suit – inch by inch – to reveal just how little you've got on underneath. He thinks you'll stop when you get to the bust, but you slowly and deliberately continue downward, unfastening each stud ultra-slowly. "I don't know how you can stand it in here, I'm almost dying of the heat," you swoon as you continue to discard your disguise...

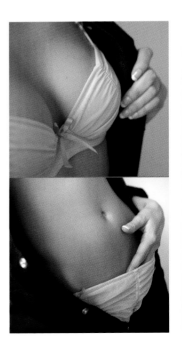

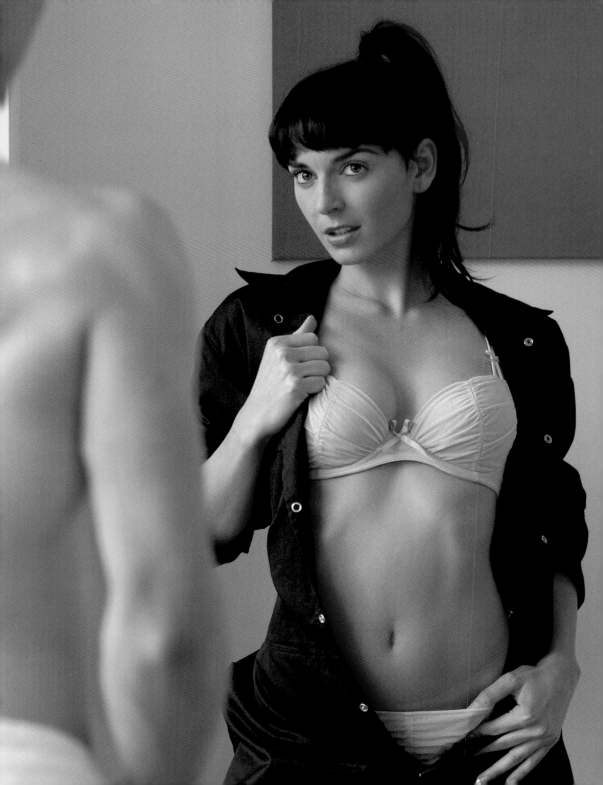

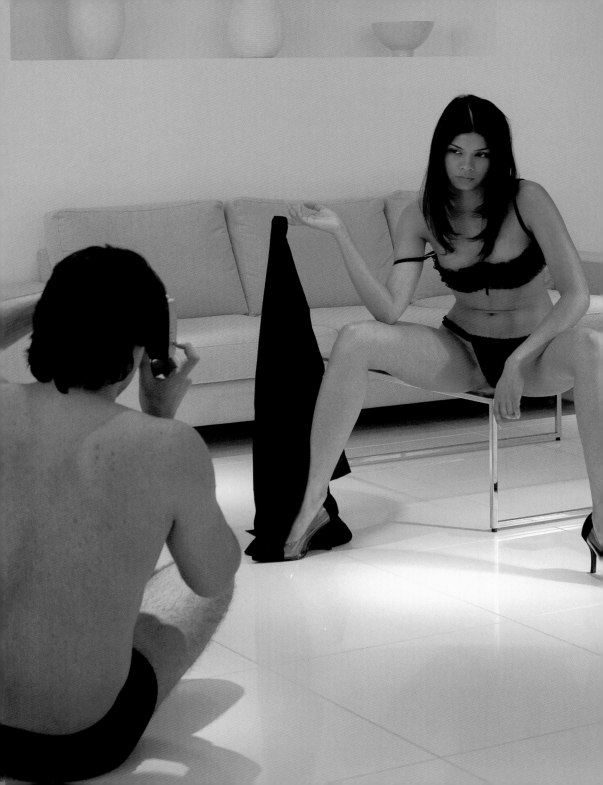

Anne's fantasy collection

There are many fascinating differences between male and female sexual fantasies. Many male fantasies, for example, are much more hard core, and this makes it difficult to fully describe them here. The following fantasies in my collection are duly modified, but you can use your imagination to work out their potential triple XXX strength and extent.

MENTAL **PREPARATION**

I feel it's important for women to understand how men's imaginations work and just how blue they can get. Many women, armed with this information, choose to alter their sexual approach, often by becoming much stronger and firmer with physical stimulation. If they're reasonably confident, they also choose to increase the games playing and fetish exploration.

THE **PORNOGRAPHER**

This fantasy involves a camera and some sexy underwear. You tell your man that he has to provide some photos for a men's magazine and that you, as the model, will assume any pose he asks for — no matter what. And then, of course, you have to provide the material he demands!

BEHIND THE **SHEET**

This sex game is inspired by one played at the annual UK rubber fetishists' ball. A small room is divided by a hanging rubber curtain, which has been coated with oil. A person on one side of the drape has no idea who is on the other side as

Anne's advice Don't think that because your man has a certain sex fantasy that you must proceed to act it out with him. In fact, most fantasies retain their power by remaining as fantasies. A fantasy is best acted out when the idea has evolved between the two of you, not just him.

they rub, stroke, and slide themselves against the body shape. In my private version of "behind the sheet," you rig up a curtain made of plastic (preferably dark and opaque), which needs to be hung securely, and cover the floor with towels. Show your partner into the room and ask him to take his clothes off and rub his body with oil. Tell him you've arranged for a friend who's a striptease artiste to visit and that you'll show her into the room shortly on the other side of the drape.

When she (you) comes into the room, he won't see who it is. To keep up the illusion, you'll need to walk in a different manner and, if you feel compelled to speak, try to disguise your voice. Once you've applied oil to yourself, start undulating against the sheet. If he doesn't move to join you, ask him to fit himself up against your body then take it from there. Even if he knows perfectly well that it's you on the other side of the curtain, the slippery sensuality of the scenario can be very erotic.

> " MANY MALE FANTASIES ARE SIGNIFICANTLY MORE HARD CORE THAN THE FEMALE VERSIONS. " *Anne*

THE **EROTIC INVENTOR**

Tell your lover that you've invented some new sex toys and you need a subject to test them on. Do this in an entirely clinical manner — you might even wear a white coat (with nothing on underneath). Having invested in an unusual collection of toys, begin the testing! Write down his comments on a pleasure scale of one to ten. When you have worked your way through the toys, select the implement that rated highest, take off your "clinic clothes," and put the star invention to full use.

Anne's advice Don't forget to oil your lover's body and genitals to facilitate the testing of your erotic inventions.

COMMON **FANTASY EXPERIENCES**

In the group A married man takes his wife to a party. As soon as they walk through the front door they realize it's not the most usual celebration. Their host is naked and, as they're ushered into the living room, they see that so too are most of the guests. "Let me take your clothes," says the host, and they feel obliged to strip. As they stand nude and vulnerable, one party guest after another walks over and starts stroking and massaging them. Eventually they're pulled over onto a huge mattress taking up at least half the room where the party continues…

Lustful female A young man from a strongly religious background describes his fantasy woman as being virtually "on heat" and willing to do almost anything to have sex with him. Sometimes she's a "bad" woman who needs correction and other times she's extremely virtuous and doing her utmost to struggle against the overwhelming sexual desire she has for this man.

The exhibitionist A man begins his sex life by making love to his girlfriend at the movies with her young brother sitting nearby and able to watch. As a married adult he imagines his beautiful wife avidly watching him making love to another woman. In the fantasy, she eventually becomes so excited she has to join in, and wife and imaginary partner are impossible to distinguish.

Sex secrets One of the major sexual differences between men and women is that men are more prone to develop fetishes, about shoes or breasts, for example. This doesn't mean they're always compelled to act on them in reality, but it does mean that fetishes can form an active part of a man's sexual imagination.

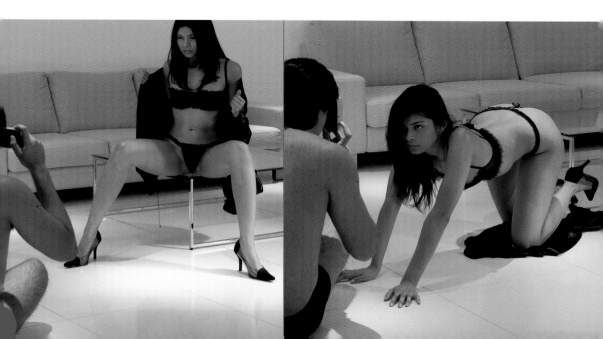

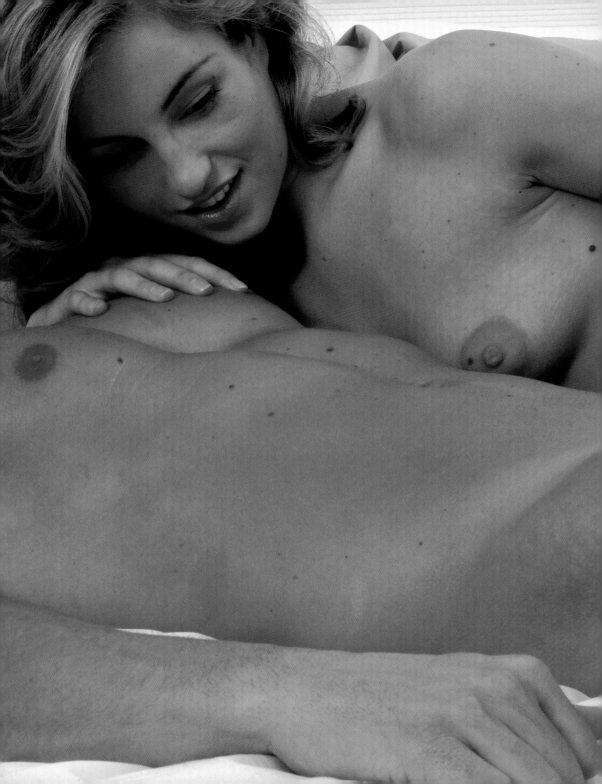

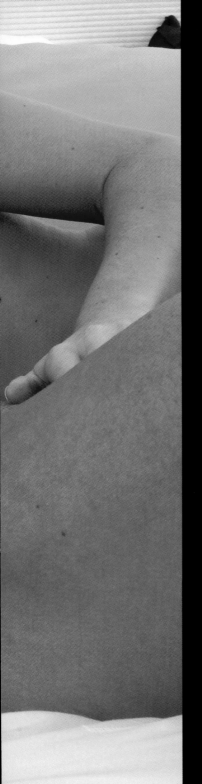

CHAPTER 6

Technical excellence

As men grow up they continue to associate physical affection with love, and if you can develop the masturbation skills described in this chapter, you will be especially emotionally valuable to your partner. As for oral sex skills, the message from the men is loud and clear. If you don't know how to do it, it's time you learned! You always have the choice of whether or not to make use of the art of fellatio, as revealed in this chapter, but if you're ignorant, the choice doesn't exist.

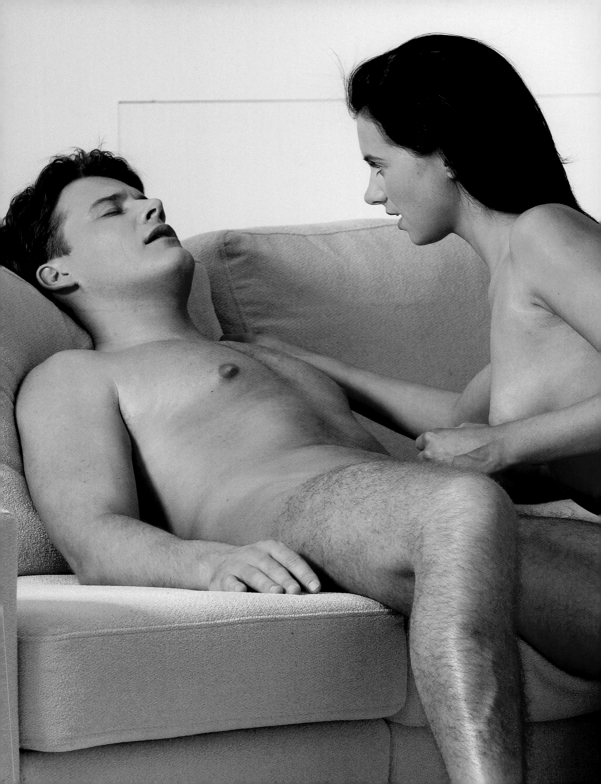

Manual stimulation

Men are sensual creatures who enjoy being made a fuss of physically. The movements, textures, or sights that create their sensual cues develop at an early age and they usually discover the good feelings associated with their penis when very young. Male self-stimulation begins in early childhood as naturally as breathing, and by the time the youngster reaches his teens he knows his sexual response in a way that many women never know theirs.

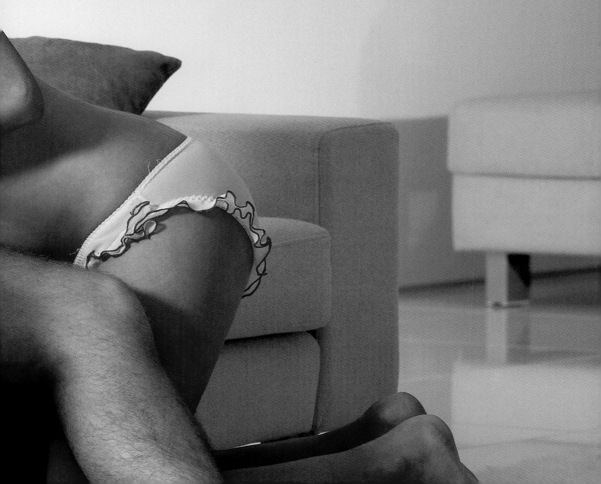

THE "MANUAL" MASSAGE

Make far more impact with a genital massage by giving a whole body massage first.

- **Aim for maximum** whole body contact.
- **Use lazy, laid-back strokes** while snuggling up against his back.
- **Stroke his abdomen** with one hand and his penis with other.
- **Slide one hand** across his chest paying special attention to his nipples while making sliding strokes on his penis.
- **Combine penis stroking** and muscle kneading along the shoulders and neck for pure sensual pleasure.

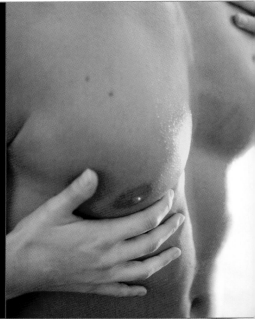

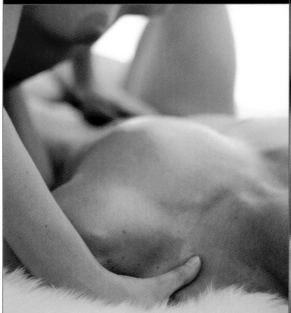

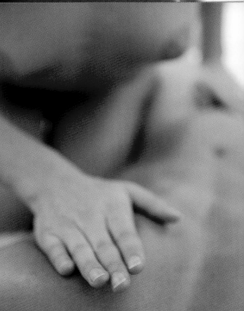

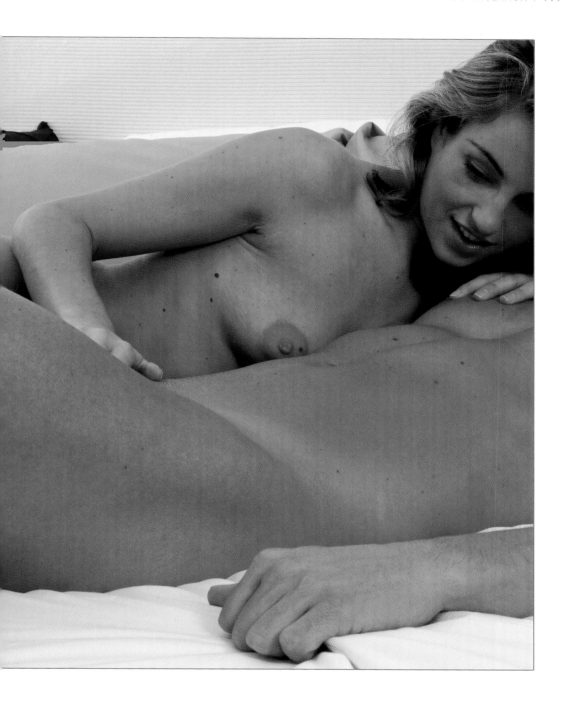

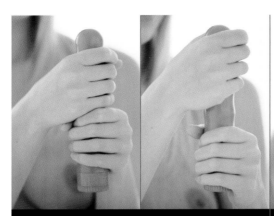

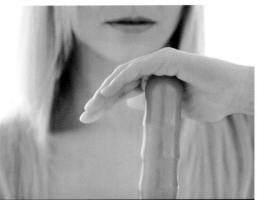

Push me-pull you Grip both hands around the middle of the penis. Then pull your hands away from each other and bring them together again repeatedly.

Juicing a lemon Grasp the penis at the base then run the palm of the other hand over and around the penis head, ten times in one direction and ten times in the other.

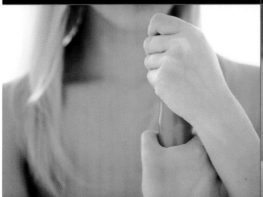

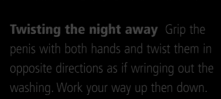

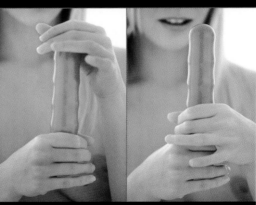

Twisting the night away Grip the penis with both hands and twist them in opposite directions as if wringing out the washing. Work your way up then down.

The rocket launch Run one grasping hand down the penis from top to bottom followed by the other. Next run one hand then the other up the penis. Repeat.

Get in training

Training in the art of masturbation is a keystone of triple XXX sex. You can use the principles and techniques during intercourse or oral sex, as well as solely for masturbation. By understanding men's genital hotspots and when and where the pressure really counts, you can excel at this much-appreciated art. But as with all art forms, perfection requires practice and this is when your vibrator gets to have some serious fun.

STAR **STROKES**

First get a life-sized vibrator or dildo to practice on (you could use a cucumber instead). You may need to steady it by wedging it into a chest of drawers and closing a drawer on it. Begin by lubricating your lucky accessory. But don't just treat him like a toy — be sensitive as you anoint him. When he is truly covered and his ridges are slipping easily through your hands, try out the star strokes opposite, which are easily the most incredible penile massage techniques that one human being can offer another. Your vibrator won't be able to give you feedback unfortunately, but at least you can get an idea of style.

If you get to be really good at your star strokes then your man may get so excited he wants to climax, and if it happens too early you might want to prevent it. If you recognize that he's getting near the point of no return, squeeze the head of the penis — on the coronal ridge — hard between finger and thumb to literally block the ducts through which the ejaculation is trying to rise (see p.80). Don't be frightened of hurting your man when doing this for real. It takes an awful lot of pressure to cause pain but it's worth putting in some secret practice on your sex toy first.

> " YOUR VIBRATOR WON'T BE ABLE TO DEMONSTRATE WHY 'THE ROCKET LAUNCH' STROKE DESERVES ITS NAME, BUT YOUR MAN PROBABLY WILL. " *Anne*

MASTERFUL MOVES

Masturbation in all its shades and variations plays a major part in male self-knowledge. One of the reasons gay couples spend so much time on whole body caressing, according to sex researchers Masters and Johnson (see p.219), is because men understand what other men secretly desire. I think it's time that women tuned into this knowledge, and being familiar with a wealth of mind-blowing masturbation moves is an excellent place to start. Below and on the next three pages is my treasure chest of male member massage methods!

Push me-pull you (see p.112) Grip both hands around the penis starting in the middle and pull your hands away from each other. Then bring them together again. These two moves in fluid repetition form the movement.

Juicing a lemon (see p.112) Grasping the penis at the base with one hand, run the palm of the other hand over and around the head of the penis, ten times in one direction and ten times in the other direction. Visually this looks as if you are juicing a lemon.

Twisting the night away (see p.112) With both hands gripped around the penis, twist them in opposite directions as if you are wringing out the washing. Then twist them the other way. Work your way up and down the shaft while doing this.

The rocket launch (see p.112) Run one gripped hand down the penis from top to bottom followed by the other. Then run first one hand then the other back up the penis. Next you run your hands down the penis twice, then back up twice. Repeat the strokes three times down and three times up, and so on all the way to ten strokes down and ten strokes up.

Anne's advice

It's essential that you have some lubricant close to hand for the real occasion, and it will help if you lubricate your lucky sex toy during training. If you rely on saliva for lubrication you can end up with an extremely dry mouth – especially if you've had wine with your dinner, which is naturally drying.

Juicing with a twist Grasp the base of the penis with one hand and using plenty of oil, rub the palm of the other hand over and around the head of the penis, rather as if you were juicing a lemon as on the previous page. This time, for even more sensation, use the hand at the base of the penis to move the penis in an opposite direction to that of your top hand. This gives an extra dimension.

The oil fall Cup your hand around his testicles with the fingers slightly spread out. Ideally the hand should be over and around the testicles rather than just underneath. With the other hand, pour some warmed oil over your hand so that it slides down your fingers and pours on to his penis and testicles. This is experienced as a kind of flooding sensation.

The slither Holding his penis at the base with one hand, use the other to encircle the top of his penis on the coronal ridge (see p.120). Turn your fingers (which have formed a ring) in a clockwise direction. When they have gone as far as they can, lift that hand slightly and, on the very head of the penis, swing your fingers back round to their starting point. Then repeat this several times.

The corkscrew Using both hands, one above the other and ringed around the penis, slowly twist your hands in opposite directions. Don't be afraid of using a firm grasp here. The contrasting strokes flood the penis with sensation.

Ring around the moon Hold the penis at the base with one hand and with the other ring the head of the penis between thumb and forefinger. Slowly and deliberately bring your "ring" up over the coronal ridge and then take it down again. As you continue with this subtle movement gradually speed it up.

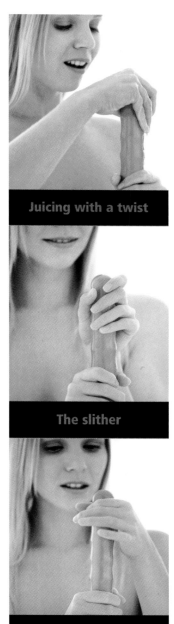

Juicing with a twist

The slither

Ring around the moon

The hand machine Hold both hands around the base of the penis with the fingers and thumbs interwoven. Then methodically raise the hands to the top of the penis, squeezing with your palms as you reach the top. Go back down again by raising the thumbs to free the penis and just let your hands slip down the penis again. Weave the thumbs together again at the bottom and go right on up again. The idea is to get a machinelike regularity of the stroke.

The heart throb Clasp both your hands around the head of the penis. Squeeze gently, and then let go. Pause and then repeat the squeeze again. The idea is to imitate the rhythm of his heartbeat. A great occasion to do this is during his ejaculation. Try and time it to his contractions, which occur at approximately 0.8 second intervals. Interestingly, the timing of male and female orgasmic contractions is identical, and the number of contractions both sexes experience during orgasm can increase with age.

The Swedish massage stroke Form rings with your fingers and thumbs and pull your ringed hands up his penis, one after the other, repeatedly. As one hand reaches the top the other is about to start pulling up at the bottom. This tends to be the way many men start off their own masturbation. An upward stroke is particularly sensational, just as it is with women's clitoral massage.

THE **STRETCHER**

First strokes The first strokes are slow and firm. Lay both your hands across the penis shaft and then move them in opposite directions so that one hand reaches the head of the penis and the other slithers right down over the testicles. You are literally stretching the penis between your hands.

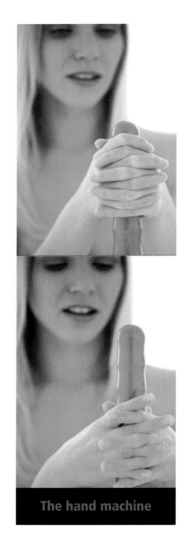

The hand machine

As you move your hands apart, slide them around so that the palms reach your man's penis extremities first.

Second strokes The second strokes are fast and light. As you reach either end of the penis, swing your hands around again so that they pivot on the head and on the testicles. Now your palms are heading back toward each other along the length of his genitals, swinging around again to the start position where they stop. Lean down above your lover while using this stroke.

Hand over hand Slide your cupped hand over the head and down the shaft of the penis. Just before your hand gets to the base, bring the other hand up to the penis head to repeat the stroke. The idea of "hand over hand" is to never let the penis remain uncovered by a moving hand.

THE **COUNTDOWN**

First strokes For the first strokes, grasp the top of his penis with your right hand and place your left hand underneath his testicles, with fingers positioned toward his anus. As you slide your right hand down his shaft, enclosing it as much as possible, bring your left hand up from his testicles. Aim to bring both hands slowly together at the base of the shaft. The countdown is rather like a reverse rocket launch (see p.114).

Second strokes Slide your right hand back up his penis from the base while simultaneously bringing your left hand back under his testicles again. As before, work slowly and steadily making the following counts:
• Ten times the first stroke, then ten times the second
• Nine times the first stroke, then nine times the second
• Eight times the first stroke, then eight times the second
• And so on, until you reach one stroke.

> " USE WARM LUBRICANT (NOT HOT) AND A STEADY BUT GENTLE PRESSURE TO ADD TO HIS PLEASURE. " *Anne*

Sex secrets Pioneer sex writer Robert Chartham suggests uncircumcised penises tend to be more sensitive than circumcised ones. This means, it's a good idea to perform your masterful moves on an uncircumcised man a little more gently.

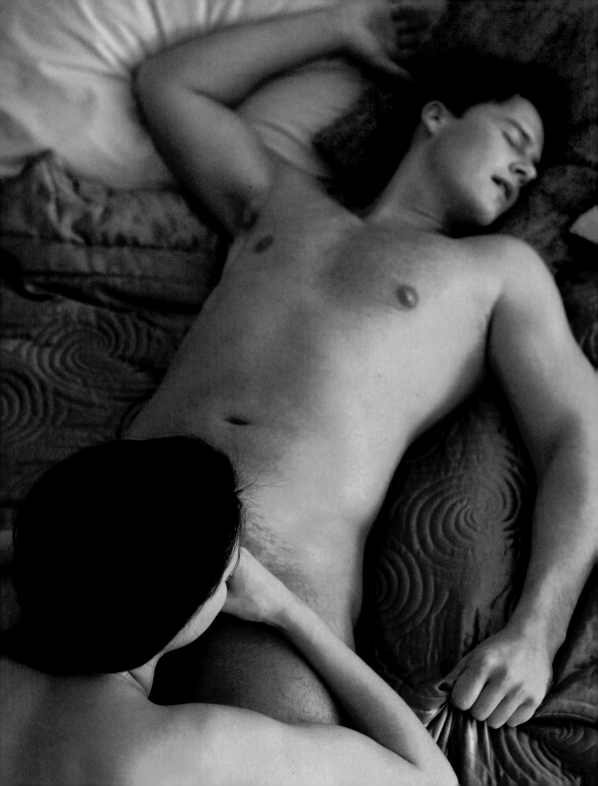

Triple XXX oral sex

My special collection of oral techniques is designed to specifically stimulate men's supersensitive zones. Many sex professionals insist that oral sex is one of the prime reasons men visit them. I see fellatio as a kind of secret weapon for women, and if you don't know how to do it well, now's your chance to learn.

AN **EXTENSION** OF **SELF**

Many men think of their penis as a separate entity to themselves, which is able take on a life of its own. It's true that you can't always control a penis. It has a slippery habit of reacting too quickly, too slowly, or of refusing to get hard when required. And yet the penis is usually seen as representative of its owner's entire sexuality. It *is* his sexuality, therefore it *is* him. This isn't logical, of course, but it means you have to be very careful how you treat your lover's genitals – you need to treat them with respect.

FELLATIO AND **MORE**

One reason that might explain why men seek sex with transsexual hookers is that these specialist sex workers possess inside knowledge of the oral stimulation that men really want. There are also certain sex positions for sexual intercourse that stimulate the supersensitive oral zones illustrated overleaf (see also p.82). The hover-fly, for example, is a woman-on-top position in which the woman raises and lowers herself rapidly on the head of her partner's penis using shallow strokes, rather than lowering herself right down. This increases sensation on the glans, frenulum, and other oral sex hotspots on the penis.

Sex secrets Linda Lovelace, the star of *Deep Throat* (a sex film made in the 1970s) is perhaps the most famous exponent of oral sex. She later told the media that she made the film against her will. As "deep throat" carries a real danger of asphyxiation for the woman, I've purposefully left this technique out of my triple XXX selection.

TRIPLE **XXX** ORAL SEX **CLASS**

It may not surprise you to realize that the penis has hot and cold spots like any other part of the body. Before you enter my triple XXX oral sex master class, I suggest you enrich your basic knowledge by learning where the penile erogenous zones are sited.

THE **SUPERSENSITIVE** PENIS

Generally, the head of the penis tends to be much more sensitive than the base. The most sensitive hot spots of all are as follows (see also p.82):

- **Glans** – the head of the penis
- **Coronal ridge** – the area just below and around the head
- **Coronal rim** – just below the ridge (a very high concentration of penile nerve endings are situated in this ridged area)
- **Frenulum** – most excitable bandlike ligament that links the coronal ridge on the underside of the penis with the penis shaft
- **Raphe** – a raised line or ridge running from the coronal ridge, down the penis, and over the middle of the testicles to the anus. This sensitive part of the male anatomy feels like a taut line running down the length of the penis.

Anne's advice The tongue is probably the most versatile sex aid we possess and, just as a pianist flexes his fingers by playing the scales before a performance, so we can train and flex our tongues. Once trained (see overleaf), the tongue can be used as a skillful tool on your lover.

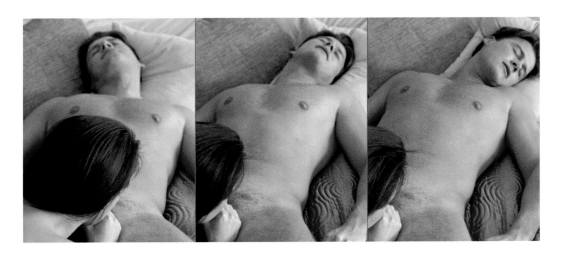

ANNE'S **RULES**

- If you feel you're being forced into performing oral sex when you don't want to, don't do it.
- If your hesitation is due to inexperience or uncertainty, try to remain open to experiment.
- If your man's penis has an unusual appearance don't blink, comment, or recoil. If it makes you happier, get to know it first. You might try this by bathing and shampooing your man (see pp.62–65). He'll love it and you'll be provided with the chance of making his intimate acquaintance.
- Don't accidentally bite your man. The best way to protect against this is to cover your teeth with your mouth so that it's your mouth that scrapes against his penis and not your teeth.
- If you don't want to swallow your man's ejaculate, never recoil from it with distaste. Many men interpret this as distaste for them personally.
- If you choose not to swallow, try to keep his ejaculate in your mouth until you can discreetly spit it out into a tissue or handkerchief kept nearby for this purpose.
- If you are a naturally dry-mouthed person, invest in some of the flavored lube capsules that have been invented especially for oral sex (see p.212). You bite on these in your mouth and they flood it with fruit-flavored gel that's harmless to ingest but which massively improves the quality of the friction your man is experiencing.
- If your man feels his sperm is inadequate, feed him tons of pumpkin seeds. These are a good source of zinc, which stimulates the hormone testosterone. This in turn affects his sperm production.
- If your man is incredibly hairy around the genitals and this seriously impedes your efforts at fellatio, don't be afraid to give him a little cosmetic grooming. After all, he gets a haircut for the top of his head regularly, doesn't he?

> " IMPROVE THE FLAVOR OF YOUR MAN'S SEMEN BY GETTING HIM TO EAT CINNAMON, NUTMEG, AND SWEET FRUIT. "
>
> *Anne*

TONGUE TRAINING
- **Sing the scales** (however badly), tonguing the word "la" very distinctly.
- **Repeat rapidly** the words, "lady," "lover," and "linguine."
- **Suck and tongue** the jam or jelly out of the center of a doughnut.
- **Buy an ice cream** cone and eat it by licking only.
- **Repeatedly push** in the buttons on your telephone with the tip of your tongue.
- **Peel a banana** and practise giving it side-to-side stimulation with the tip of your tongue.

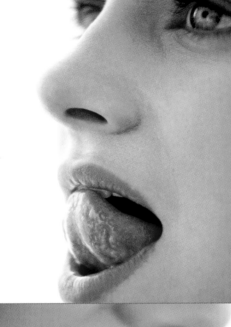

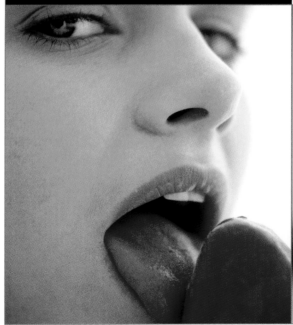

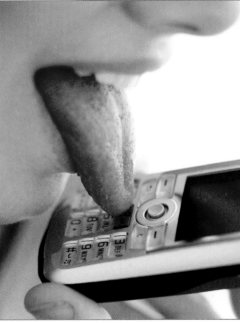

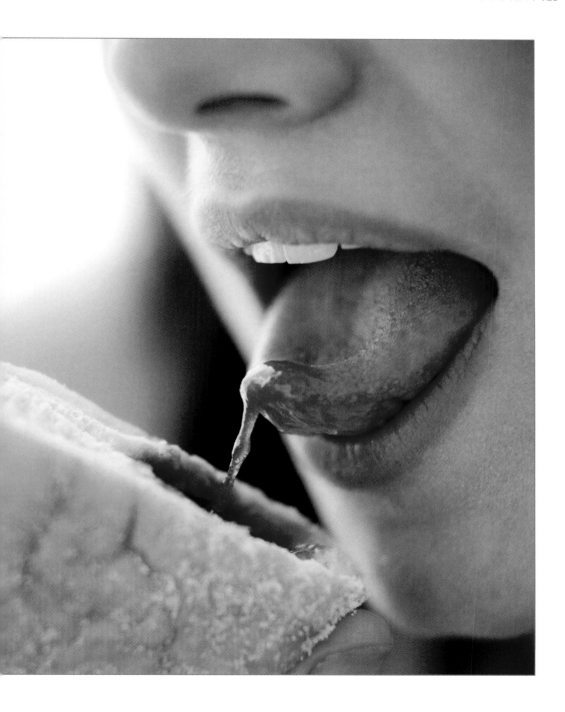

Mouth movements

The next step in my triple XXX oral sex master class is to develop an appreciation of the variety of pressures that you can incorporate into your repertoire of fellatio using your lips, mouth, and tongue.

DELICIOUS **VARIETY**

- **Sensual suction** There's an art to sucking a penis, which can only really be mastered with practice. Judicious sucking is best. It's a bad idea to vacuum your man so hard that he emerges with bruises – a less forceful suction is recommended. You can suck on the whole head of his penis or focus on sucking your way up and down the shaft.
- **The flat sword** This is an upward tongue movement in which you lick your way up your man's penis with a broad, pointed (or sword-shaped) tongue. You can begin at the base of the penis, or even on or behind the testicles. The movement must be upward because this gives more sensation than a downward movement.
- **Glossy lips** Coat your lips with saliva or tasteless lubricating gel and with your lips planted firmly on the penis, push them up and down without losing any contact with the skin.
- **Mouth vibration** Pucker your lips close together and then force air out between them, as if you were blowing a raspberry without using your tongue. Try doing this at regular intervals with your mouth hard up against your man's penis. You're bound to make quite an impact.
- **Humming bird** With his penis enclosed in your mouth, hum while sliding your mouth up and down him. The vibrations of your humming sound reverberate up and down his shaft.

Sex secrets Kenneth Ray Stubbs recommends using "daisy kisses" (whole mouth kisses with just a little bit of suction) to cover your partner's entire body before applying them solely to his penis.

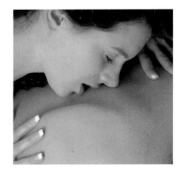

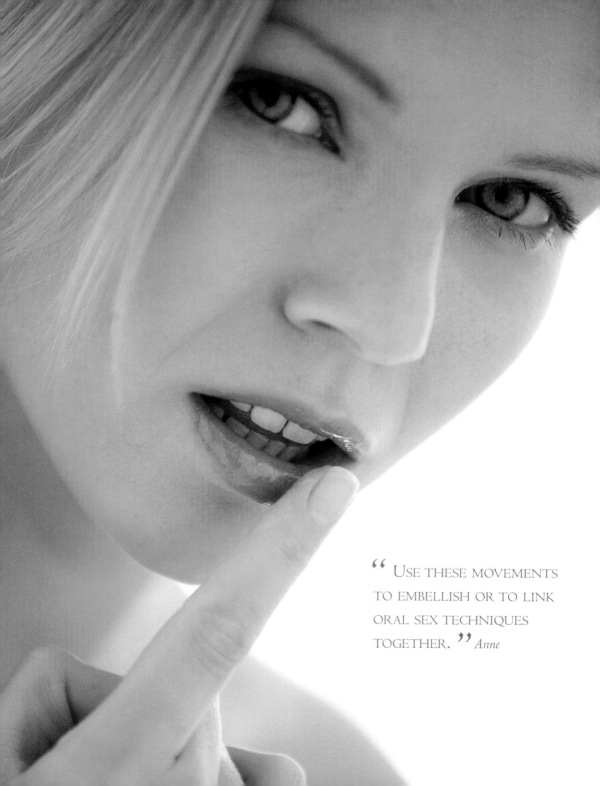

" Use these movements to embellish or to link oral sex techniques together. " *Anne*

A **HELPING HAND**

Your hands can do so much more than merely act as stabilizers while your mouth gives your man's penis all the attention. The dual action of hand and mouth gives the delightful impression that your man has, not one, but two women working on him.

The butterfly flick Holding the penis base steady with one hand, take the penis head in your mouth. As your mouth moves up and down, flicker your tongue rapidly backward and forward across the frenulum (see p.82). As this area is highly sensitive, the technique may be best left until the end of the proceedings.

Lip synching Make a ring around the top of his penis using your thumb and fingers, then keep the "ring" firmly against

Sex secrets According to the famous madam Xaviera Hollander (see p.218), tongue "strumming" (which entails fast, rhythmical flickering of the tongue against the penis) is the single most important skill a woman should excel at if she wants to be outstandingly good at fellatio.

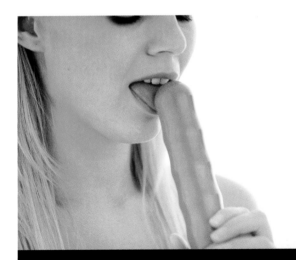

The butterfly flick As your mouth moves up and down his penis, flicker your tongue backward and forward across the frenulum.

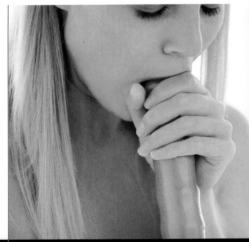

Lip synching Make a ring around the pe with your thumb and fingers and hold it ne to your mouth as you move up and down.

your mouth as you move your mouth up and down his penis. With your thumb and fingers "attached" to your lips, it feels to him as if your mouth has grown an extension. In his mind you have the longest mouth ever to offer fellatio.

Twist and shout You twist. He shouts. As your mouth moves up and down his penis and your left hand holds him steady at the base, your right hand slides and twists around the shaft. He feels two distinctly different moves simultaneously.

Tongue sculpting Holding the base of his penis with both hands, use the broad blade of your tongue as a sculpting tool to push his penis around and about as you shape him up. This is a good technique to use when your man is flaccid.

Anne's advice As you draw your mouth up from your man's penis, try pulling down the hand holding the penis until the skin is stretched quite hard against your mouth. This makes the sensitive ending of the penis taut and more exposed.

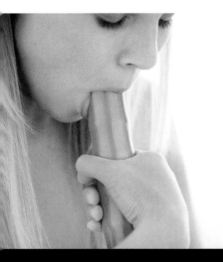

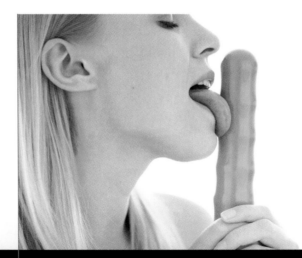

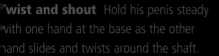

Twist and shout Hold his penis steady with one hand at the base as the other hand slides and twists around the shaft.

Tongue sculpting Holding the penis base steady with both hands, use the broad blade of your tongue to lick him into life.

Tricks and treats

Like every other aspect of sex, fellatio benefits from skillful use of the imagination. I've already indicated that surprise plays a key part in sexual arousal. This is because anything that gives you a "jolt" raises your adrenaline levels — and this, in turn, affects the cells in the brain responsible for sexual response. Here are some simple tricks for making oral sex an extraordinary treat and getting his arousal rates soaring.

MAGIC MOMENTS

Lemon sherbet Suck on one of these tangy sweets before taking him in your mouth. The surprisingly intense fizzing and bursting sensation that sherbet gives off feels quite extraordinary on the supersensitive skin of the penis.

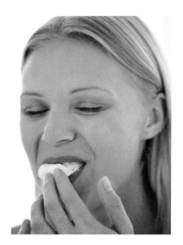

Marshmallow moments Before beginning oral sex, fill your mouth up with two or three marshmallow cubes. The sensation for him is like thrusting into a cloud — but a cloud with extra texture that feels amazing.

Ice cubes and hot tea This game of heat contrast depends on having the necessary ingredients prepared ahead and close at hand. Begin by filling your mouth with ice cubes before sucking on your man. After a short time, get rid of the ice and take a couple of gulps of hot tea, making sure that your mouth heats up properly. Then take your man back into your mouth. The best way to make this work is to do it as fast as possible so that he experiences the extreme contrasts of heat and cold rapidly.

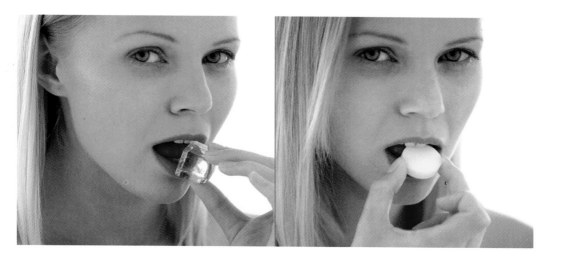

Toothpaste tingle Toothpaste is a magic ingredient for creating oral sex treats – simply rinse a little around your mouth before oral sex. "Toothpaste tingle," however, can feel pretty sharp so don't overdose on it.

Mint mouthwash For this less intense version of toothpaste tingle, simply rinse the mint mouthwash around your mouth before going down.

Suck on a strong mint Perhaps your partner actually enjoys a little masochism. A strong mint may well be too much for some, but occasionally your man may crave a really intense experience.

Tantalizing his testicles Many women don't realize how sensitive the male testicles can be. Check your man's sensitivity by taking each of his testicles in your mouth and slowly passing your tongue underneath each one, letting the sacs slip gently across your mouth.

" A BURST OF ADRENALINE CAUSED BY UNEXPECTED SENSATIONS HEIGHTENS SEXUAL PERCEPTION IN THE BRAIN. " *Anne*

Anne's advice Try taking as much of his testicles into your mouth as you can, then hum a tune while simultaneously tongue flicking. Rachmaninov does it for my partner, or you could go for the yogic chant of "om."

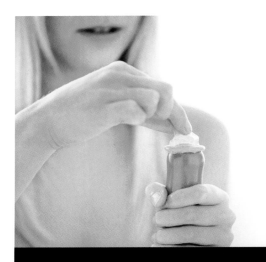

Squeeze out air Gently press the tip of
the condom to ensure it contains no air.

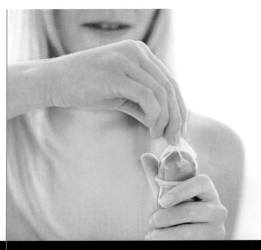

Keep squeezing as you position the
condom. An air bubble can cause a split.

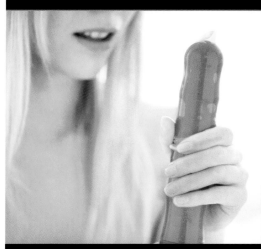

Begin to roll Once the condom is
covering the head begin to roll it down.

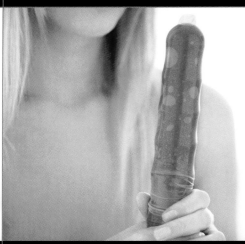

A secure fit Roll the condom right
down to bottom of the penis shaft.

The erotic condom

Unless you know absolutely for certain that your lover is a virgin it's a good idea to use condoms, even for oral sex. There's an amazing Thai method for putting on condoms with the mouth so that his penis cladding feels to a man like part of the natural process of lovemaking. Getting your condom clothing technique perfect can take some practice, however, and your man's erection may not be the best place to begin. You could try out your skills on a life-sized vibrator first!

CONDOM **ROLLING**

Practice condom rolling on your favorite vibrator (or a "penis-sized" cucumber may do just as well). Hold the unrolled sheath by the tip, squeezing it so that no air can be trapped as an air bubble can be risky. If you put pressure on it during intercourse the condom is capable of splitting.

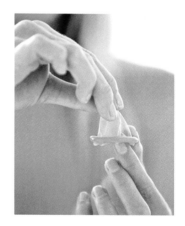

Holding your vibrator near the head, place the sheath on the tip and, with your hand slightly curved, just smooth it on and down, trying to make the move a continuous smoothing motion. Your vibrator has the advantage of possessing a permanent erection. Your man does not. This means that his erection will need to be encouraged before it will be possible to place a condom on him during the real event. Practicing your technique for rolling by hand first gives you a very good idea of the way condoms can be maneuvered and can make using them a seamless and sensuous affair.

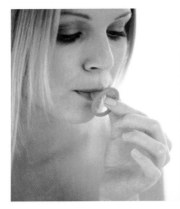
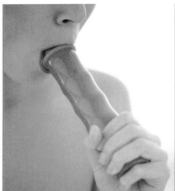
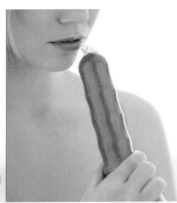

THE **MOUTH MAESTRO**

After practicing rolling a condom by hand, practice rolling one on using your mouth. Close your mouth tight on the tip of a condom and, as you hold the base of the vibrator steady with one hand, let your mouth push the condom down onto the vibrator as it rises up into your mouth. Cover your teeth with the rim of your mouth so there's no risk of nicking the condom. Simply push slowly down onto the vibrator until you have gone as far as you can go without gagging. You can use your tongue to smooth it down if this helps. If you can't get the sheath far enough down, don't be afraid of letting your fingers take over from your mouth. But the idea is to make the process a continuous and flowing one. Practice until perfect.

TESTING TIME

Finally, you might want to double check how well you've rolled your condom. All this attention you've given your vibrating friend may have made you feel horny. Here's where you insert the freshly sheathed sex toy into your vagina and exercise your vaginal muscles on it. If, after some racy treatment, your toy still retains his overcoat, then you've passed the class with honors. Now you're ready for the real man.

Anne's advice

Customers of Thai condom rolling experts say they can't tell the difference between a penis mouth massage and being condom clad. This may reflect an insensitivity on their part, but the message is that the donning of a condom can be made to feel genuinely like a part of lovemaking.

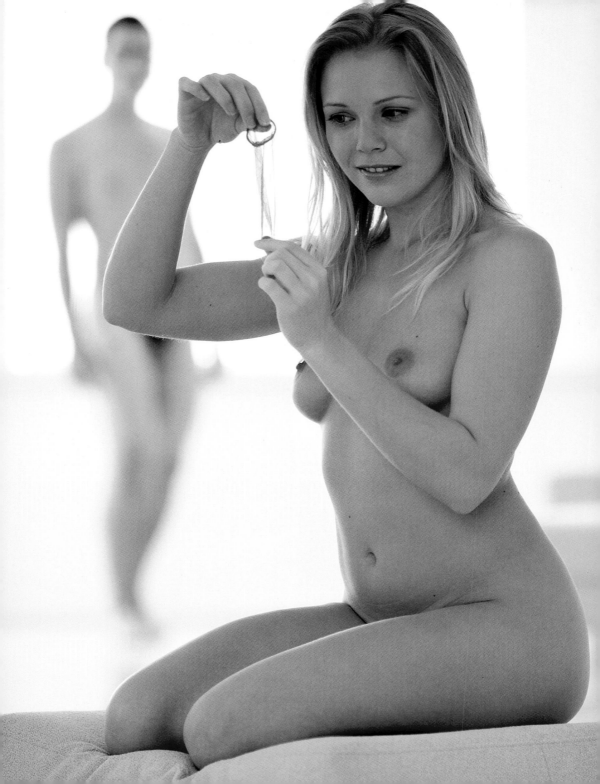

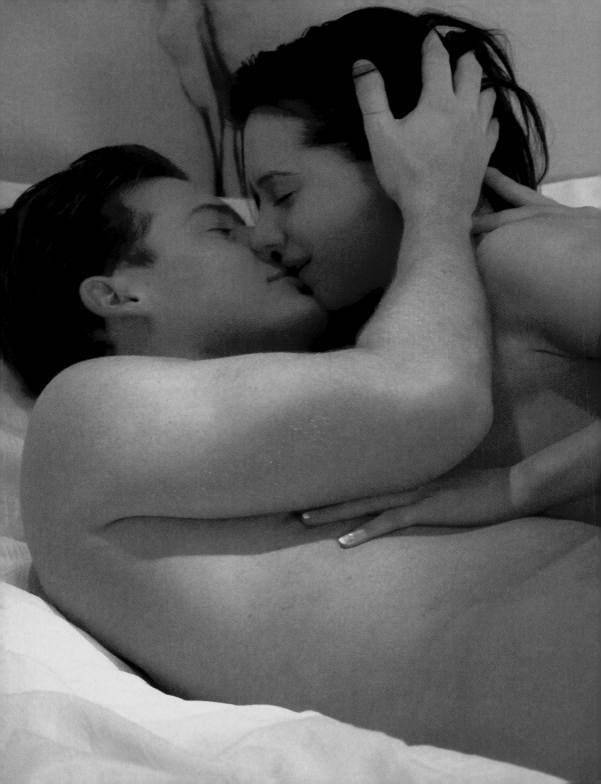

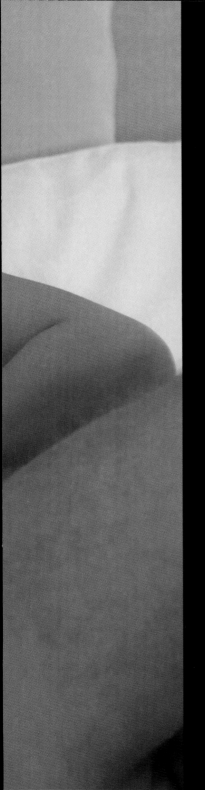

CHAPTER 7

The unexpected

This chapter focuses on one of the best kept sex secrets of all time, concerning a taboo part of the male body. So if you think you'll be shocked, turn straight to page 142 and don't collect an unexpected pleasure experience on the way! But if you're feeling curious, adventurous, and willing to learn (if not try out) something special, then read on. And if you're still wondering: "P" stands for pleasure and also for prostate, as in the explosively sensitive prostate gland.

Opening up the rosebud

The prostate is a small gland located at the top of the anal passage that feels like a bump. It's this gland that's responsible for manufacturing seminal fluid – the secretion that sweeps your man's sperm off on the journey to find an egg. What isn't mentioned in the biology textbooks is that this gland can be the source of extraordinary sexual pleasure.

ASSESS YOUR MAN

The first question to ask is does your man actually want prostate massage? There are many men who would consider any exploration of their "forbidden zone" to be a fate worse than death. If your guy's one of these, you'd be wise to move on and ignore the temptations outlined here. You can find out by moving a playful finger near his derrière and watching his reaction. If he roughly pushes you away, that's a clear message. If he looks strangely passive and gives the impression that he's waiting for more, then he probably is…waiting for more.

HOW TO PROCEED?

Don't feel obliged to try any prostate massage if you're not comfortable – you must make a completely free choice. And you don't have to "delve in" as far as his prostate if it feels difficult or awkward. If you are interested but uncertain, you could start by stroking the highly sensitive entrance to the anal passage. Anal "bathing" is always your starting point no matter how far you intend to go. Very short fingernails are a prerequisite, and because the anal area has no natural lubrication you will need a good gooey lubricant. You could try anal stimulation on yourself first to get an idea of sensation and method.

> " THE ENTIRE ANAL REGION IS LADEN WITH SENSITIVE NERVE ENDINGS, AND THE P-SPOT IS THE MOST DYNAMIC AREA OF ALL. " *Anne*

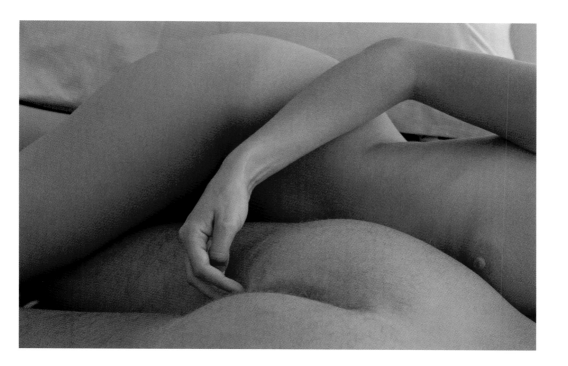

THE **ROSEBUD MASSAGE**

- **Begin by massaging** the outer region of the anus. Using a gentle pressure, run a well lubricated finger around the outside of the "rosebud."
- **Next insert your finger** slightly and gently run it around the inside of the anus. This is called "rimming."
- **As you rim**, push against the outer entrance as if you are trying to open his rosebud. You're gently stretching him.
- **Stretch him enough** to get two fingers inside him. Then slide two slightly curved fingers in and out, moving from the front to the back of his body. (The sites at the front and back are where the most nerve endings lie, as opposed to the sides.)
- **Slide your fingers** in and out by about an inch (2cm) without withdrawing your fingers completely. You could use a rocking motion once you gain confidence.

Anne's advice Before venturing into this "forbidden" new territory, immaculate hygiene is a must. Any sex acts involving the anal passage should only be considered after a shower, bath, or bidet.

The P-spot

The P-spot can be considered to be the male equivalent of the female G-spot. 'P' stands for the male prostate gland, located at the top of the anal passage on the upper side (nearest his belly). This hidden pleasure zone tends to be overlooked by both sexes, which is a pity because massage of the prostate alone can bring a man to orgasm.

HITTING THE SPOT

This is where it helps to have long fingers. The P-spot (prostate gland) is located on the uppermost side at the far end of the anal passage at an approximate 12 o'clock position. When his "rosebud" feels receptive, slide your finger up the anal passage and try to locate the prostate "bump." Be very careful about your fingernails — they must be short and smooth. You may prefer to wear a close-fitting latex glove as an extra safeguard, but with or without a glove, your finger must be well lubricated.

P IS FOR PLEASURE

1 In order to give his anal sphincter time to adapt, take your finger insertion in stages. Halt every so often until his muscles have sufficiently relaxed. Be warned; these stops may need to be for as long as a minute.

2 By the time your whole finger has penetrated him, you're nearing the P-spot. When you find it, try stroking it with a slightly curved finger as if you are beckoning, over and over again. Don't let your nail make contact with the surface. It's the softness of your finger pad that's needed here.

3 If you can sustain this movement, it's highly likely to send him mad with pleasure.

Anne's advice You can feel the prostate gland as a firm, walnut-sized "bump." By pressing it in a sustained, regular rhythm you can provide your partner with a great deal of unexpected pleasure.

4 When your stimulation is no longer needed, withdraw very slowly. Give his anal passage a chance to relax again after the contractions of orgasm.

TOYS FOR BOYS...AND OTHER PLOYS

Many women find that their fingers are too short to reach as far as the P-spot. This is where sex toys make a spectacular *aide digitale* (see also pp.204–205). The wonder sex toy of all time, the vibrator, comes in special designs for anal use. P-spot vibrators are slimmer than the vaginal cigar-shaped ones, they bulge slightly in the middle, and have a small hilt at the end. The slimness is to make anal penetration easy, the bulge is to hold the vibrator in place once it has moved up the anus, and the hilt is to ensure that it doesn't travel too far inside. The newest varieties work with pulsation, not just vibration, which is especially stimulating for the P-spot.

> " IT'S THOUGHT THAT THE P-SPOT SHARES THE SAME DEVELOPMENTAL ORIGINS AS THE FEMALE G-SPOT. "
> *Anne*

HOW TO REACH HIS P-SPOT

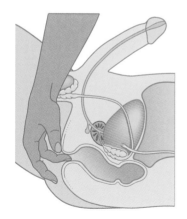

The prostate gland encircles the urethra at the exit from the bladder.

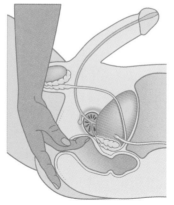

Insert a well lubricated finger into his anus and press against the front wall.

P-SPOT **PLUGS**

Plugs can be used as a stimulant, to train the anal passage, and to offer feelings of fullness. They're sometimes used in games of domination or by those who want extra anal stimulation during masturbation. Plugs come in a number of sizes and materials.

ANAL **BEADS**

These comprise a string of connected plastic beads — a bit like old-fashioned "poppets" that can't be pulled apart. Once the beads have been skillfully pressed into your man's anus, they are pulled out while he is having his orgasm. This carefully timed bonus seriously increases his climatic sensation.

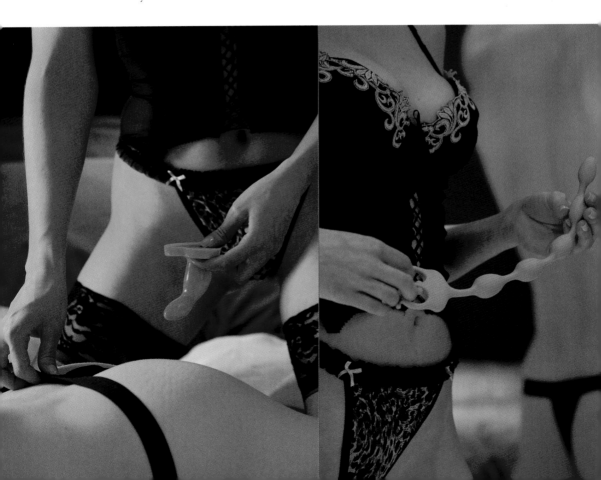

TOY TIPS

- **All sex toys** used for P-spot play need to be scrupulously cleaned before reuse. (You may be encouraged to know, however, that a recently emptied bowel contains less bacteria than the inside of a human mouth!)
- **Clothing your sex toys** in condoms or other latex is unsexy, but it does reduce the risk of sexually transmitted disease.
- **Check any plastic** sex toys for rough edges. If there are any, file them down with a metal nail file. It's imperative that penetrative objects are smooth.
- **Remember you should never** have vaginal intercourse directly after anal intercourse without washing first.

" KENNETH RAY STUBBS SUGGESTS COMBINING ANAL STIMULATION WITH INTERCOURSE. YOU NEED TO BE A BIT OF A CONTORTIONIST, BUT I PROMISE YOU IT'S POSSIBLE! " *Anne*

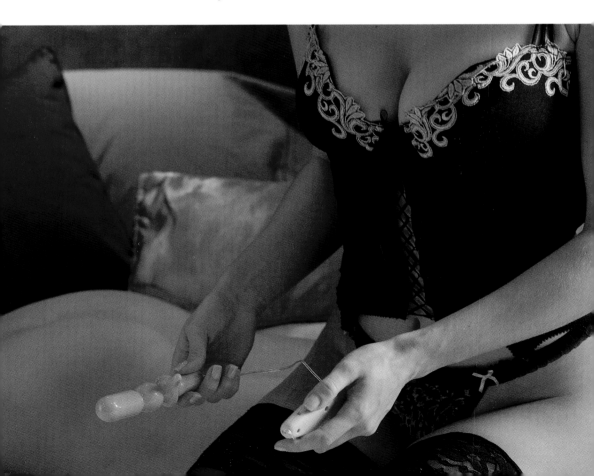

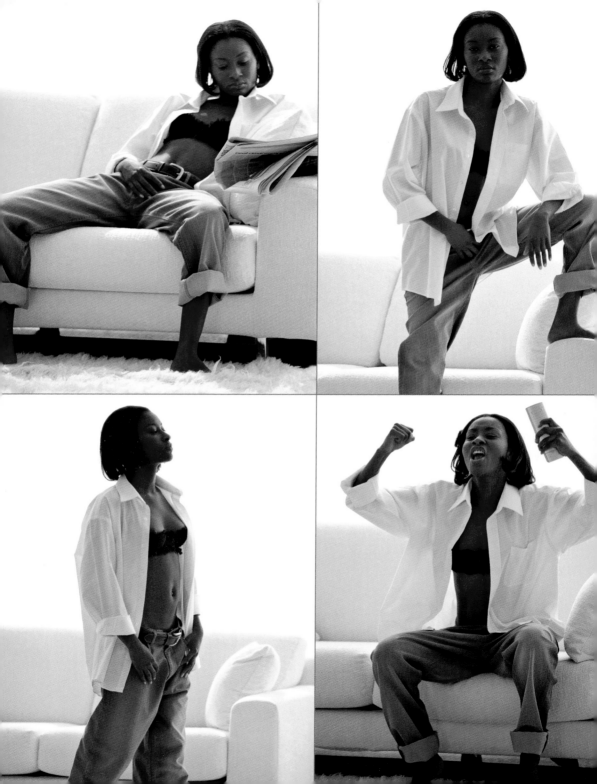

Explore your inner man

A novel concept has developed called the Drag King Workshop. Drag King Dianne Torr (see p.219) holds such workshops all over North America and Europe. Women of all ages, religions, and ethnic groups attend Dianne's seminars to get in touch with their masculine side.

HOW TO BE A DRAG KING

- **Imagining** Lower your voice and slow things down. Imagine what kind of man you are and who your male role model is.
- **Sitting** Sit with your legs wide apart and your feet flat on the ground. Read a newspaper or rest your hands on your "penis."
- **Standing up** Take your time. Lean forward and stand up straight before then taking a step.
- **Walking** The action comes from the top half of the body. Your weight falls first to one side then the other — the hips don't wiggle. Make longer strides than you would normally, and tough luck to anyone who blunders into your personal space.
- **Gesturing** Gestures are decisive and strong. You might, for example, punch the air.

> " BEHAVIOR YOU FELT YOU COULD NEVER PARTICIPATE IN AS CATHY, IS EASILY ACCESSIBLE AS BILL. "
> *Dianne Torr*

MALE INSIGHTS

So what's the point of you, a heterosexual woman, putting on male clothes and parading as a man? The brief answer is that it allows you to gain a real insight into what it's like to be a man. You learn how it feels physically and you can see how other people perceive you as a man (which is very different from how they perceive you as a woman). This gives you an extremely useful insight into your man's inner desires, and your new sense of "masculinity" may lend power to your everyday behavior.

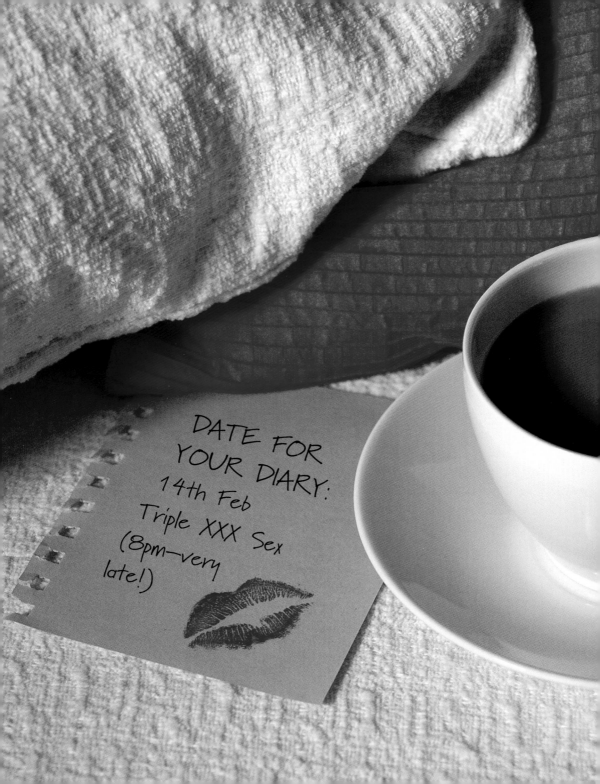

Unexpected surprises

Many sex educators recommend devising small surprises for your lover to keep the adrenaline rising in established relationships. I've practiced doing this myself with very pleasing results. You could try tucking a suggestive note under the windscreen wiper on his car or leaving your shopping list out where he can't fail to see it on which a key item reads, "Sex with ..." (write his name in the gap).

NOVELTY VERSUS FAMILIARITY

Couples who complain that sex is boring are often asked by their therapists to make love the next time doing something fractionally different, such as lying on the side of the bed that your partner normally occupies. What therapists like me are aiming to do is to bring novelty into the equation, even if it involves making tiny changes. If making love with the left hand instead of the right hand, for example, doesn't feel right, then that's good, believe it or not. It means your brain is registering something different and this is the beginning of change.

INTRODUCING CHANGE

Sex, like anything else, can become routine. It's often an extremely pleasurable routine that has evolved for a good reason – because it works. But you have laid down a pattern in the brain, literally, that can be hard to shift. Some men don't want to shift at all and are very resistant to attempts at change. For them routine is the way to have sex and they get angry when you aim at something else. So don't try the suggestion on the next page unless you're sure it'll be appreciated...

Anne's advice Not all surprises are welcome. I know of one man who, when presented with airline tickets for a sexy weekend, shut himself in his apartment for three days while his girlfriend went away with her mother. The moral? It pays to know your man before plotting and scheming.

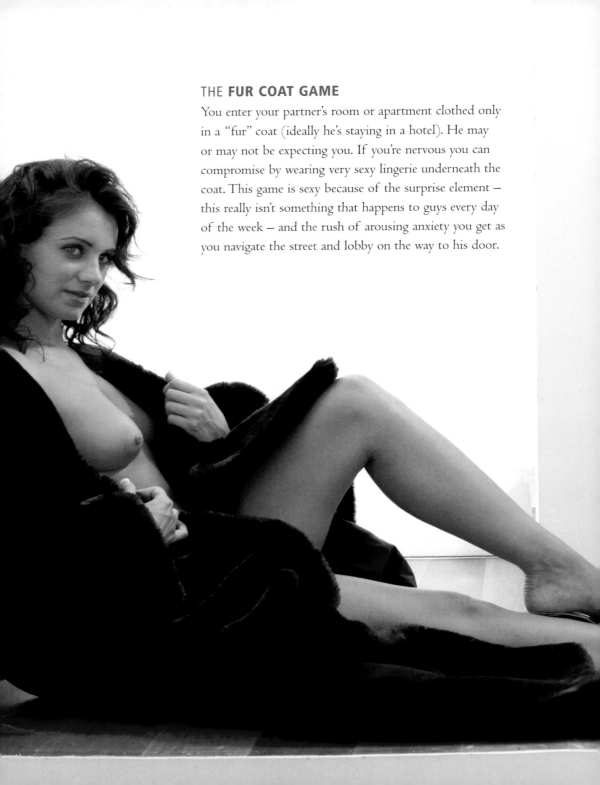

THE **FUR COAT GAME**

You enter your partner's room or apartment clothed only in a "fur" coat (ideally he's staying in a hotel). He may or may not be expecting you. If you're nervous you can compromise by wearing very sexy lingerie underneath the coat. This game is sexy because of the surprise element — this really isn't something that happens to guys every day of the week — and the rush of arousing anxiety you get as you navigate the street and lobby on the way to his door.

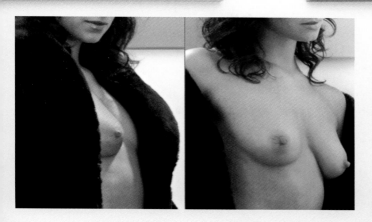

“ THE BEST UNEXPECTED SURPRISE
I EVER MANAGED TO GIVE TO A
LOVER WAS THE FUR COAT GAME
— IT WORKED BRILLIANTLY! ” *Anne*

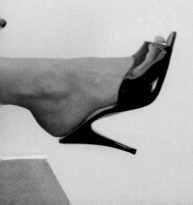

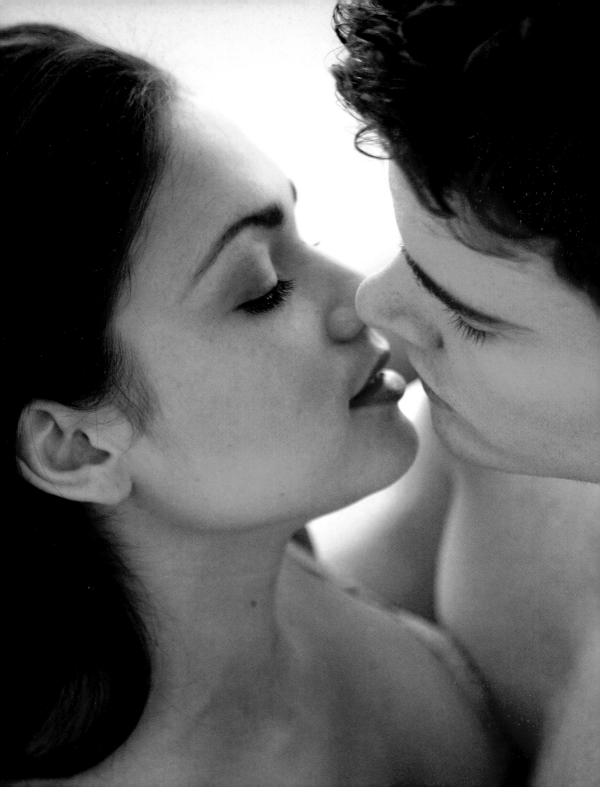

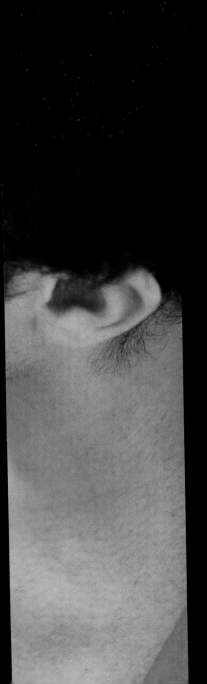

CHAPTER 8

The spiritual side of sex

Long before the advent of
Christianity, men and women
attained a godlike state through
lovemaking. Masculinity was thought
to be a source of spiritual power
and strength, and a woman in love
adored her man as if he were a god.
We may dismiss such concepts
as meaningless today, but should
you consider putting some of the
spiritual precepts in this chapter into
practice, you might see your man
grow perceptibly in self-esteem and
loving behavior.

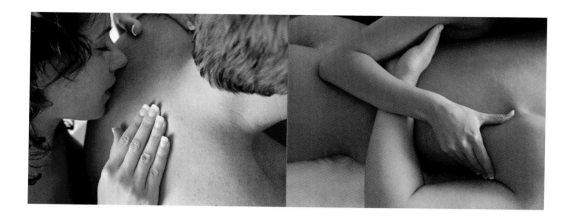

Pathway of extreme pleasure

Way before Christianity took hold in the West, a key to spiritual fulfillment was thought to lie within the ecstasy of the sex act. I believe that by evoking powerful sex sensations you can increase your spirituality, and this can be encouraged via two separate pathways. The first is the pathway of extreme sexual pleasure, detailed here, and the second is the pathway of loving intimacy (see pp.156–157).

SENSITIZING PLEASURE SPOTS

Kenneth Ray Stubbs (see p.219) is one of the few sex educators who brings spirituality into his workshops and books. One of several techniques he endorses is that of sensitizing pleasure spots. Here are the "secret" erogenous zones that he taught the students of the National Sex Forum massage classes, plus one of my own additions. Have these in mind as you embark upon your pathway of sexual pleasure.

Neck spots Many of us will have discovered this by accident when our lover adoringly kisses or bites us around the ear, neck, and shoulder. It's an area so sensitive that it affects arousal throughout the body, especially the genitals. To find it, look at the base of your man's head, where the back of the skull meets the top of the neck. Directly underneath the skull, on either side of the neck vertebrae, you will find some small muscles, which may feel very tight. This area is a secret sensation source that responds to massaging or "thrumming."

Shoulder blades Crook your partner's arm across and up his back. This lifts his shoulder blade so that you can lightly massage underneath it. Some people have an extreme sensation spot in this area.

Inner pelvis Gently press into the areas where his legs meet the front of his pelvis using both hands on both sides of the pelvis simultaneously. Start at the bottom of these areas and gently work your way up about 2 inches (6cm). You're looking for the places where prominent, ropelike ligaments (inguinal ligaments) cross from the pelvis to the legs. Press gently in and rotate on and around these ligaments without moving your fingers across the skin surface.

Penile base Following a sensual massage (including a genital one), locate the area where your partner's scrotal sac begins underneath the penis. Pushing gently but firmly, feel the base of the penis through the sac and then rotate the skin beneath your fingers across the penis shaft. Simultaneously massage the top of the penis with your other hand. As most men don't massage the base of the penis during masturbation, the sensation should be a new one. The combination of strokes gives the impression that all parts of the genitals are being stroked.

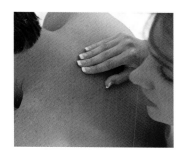

Anne's advice Ask someone to stimulate your neck spots to understand how best to massage your partner's. Go in lightly. Too much pressure on this sensitive area can hurt.

" THE PAGAN IDEA OF DERIVING ALMOST GODLIKE STATURE FROM A HAPPY ENJOYMENT OF LOVEMAKING IS NOT SUCH A BAD ONE! " Anne

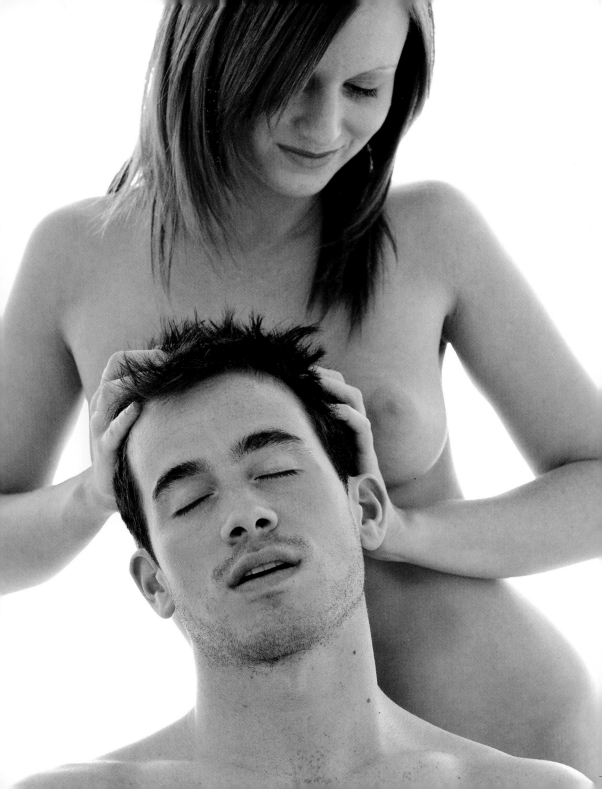

Spiritual massage

Indian head massage is an ancient Indian treatment that relieves tension and stress in the shoulders, neck, scalp, and face. It also improves the circulation in the brain and enhances the senses. Traditionally carried out fully clothed, this version is conducted in the nude and makes the recipient both relaxed and alert – a perfect combination for great sex.

THE **SEQUENCE**

Get your partner to sit up straight in a chair and gently place your hands on the crown of his head. Using your palms and fingertips rub the head, going from the sides and back up to the crown. Then use your fingertips and thumbs to press on the scalp in a downward and forward movement, creating heat through friction with small, rhythmic movements. Work your way like this over the entire head then follow these steps:

1 Place the heels of your hands over his temples and, keeping one hand still, vigorously move the other hand up and down on the same spot. Repeat this step using the other hand.
2 Very gently pull the hair at the sides of his head and rub the areas in front and above the ears using a circular motion.
3 Place your fingers pointing upward on both temples and repeatedly squeeze inward for five seconds then release.
4 Rub the small muscles on either side of his neck firmly then tilt his head back and rest it on your thumbs for fifteen seconds.
5 Knead the trapezius muscles across the tops of his shoulders to relax the base of the neck and shoulder area.
6 Finally, awaken his senses by lightly bouncing your fingertips over the head, "plucking" the hair as you go.

> " INDIAN HEAD MASSAGE ("CHAMPI" IN HINDI) STEMS FROM AN INDIAN TRADITION OF FAMILY GROOMING THAT'S OVER A THOUSAND YEARS OLD. " *Anne*

Fire breath orgasm

This Native American shamanic tradition has been resurrected by Harley Swiftdeer in the US. According to Harley, fire breath orgasms formed part of traditional Cherokee ceremonies because they enabled the Cherokees to sense the forces of creation, which rushed through them during energizing climaxes. In a modern context, these techniques (which can be used by both men and women) can reinvigorate sexual energy and enable orgasms to be experienced more profoundly.

HOW TO **EXPERIENCE** A **FIRE BREATH** ORGASM

1 Lie down on a firm surface.

2 Relax and let go of tension.

3 Take deeper breaths, inhaling through the nose and exhaling through the mouth.

4 As you continue this breathing, rock your pelvis so that you tilt it forward on the inhale and rock it backward on the exhale.

5 Once you've got this routine moving regularly, squeeze your vaginal or penile muscles on the exhale (as if you were trying to prevent the flow of urine) and at the same time flatten your back. These synchronized movements stimulate sensation in the genitals.

6 As you inhale, imagine you are filling your stomach with air and letting it out like a balloon. Repeat this continuously.

7 As this routine becomes comfortable, let your knees open and close like "quivering flames."

8 Now begin to visualize energy growing like waves of heat across different parts of your body. As you pull in the air

" FIRE BREATH ORGASMS CLEAR THE BODY OF OLD HURTS AND HELP PRE-ORGASMIC WOMEN BECOME GENITALLY ORGASMIC. "

Annie Sprinkle

from the atmosphere you are sending it down to your central-lower body area. Begin by sending it to your perineum (the area between the penis or vagina and the anus). Visually circulate the energy here. When you feel that the area is heating up, repeat this in the stomach region, then circulate the heated air from the stomach to the perineum and back again.

9 Next circulate the heated air from the stomach to the heart, backward and forward as before.

10 Now circulate the heated air from the heart to the throat. Don't worry if you find you're making sounds involuntarily while doing this. The sounds help open up the throat to the circulating energy.

11 Next move the air circulation from the throat to the "third eye" (the area in the middle of the forehead).

12 Then move the energy from the third eye to the top of the head. At a certain stage you may feel as if the energy is roaring out of the top of your head. Your breathing pattern will probably have become much faster and shallower. This is the point at which some people are able to experience the fire breath orgasm. And it's an orgasm that stretches on for an exceptionally long time!

Don't worry if you don't experience orgasm. What really counts is that the breathing experience clears the body of energetic "blockages." These blockages might be past experiences that inhibit you or hold you back. You can practice fire breath techniques during intercourse. The techniques have been known to improve orgasm and to enable people to experience orgasm during intercourse for the first time.

It really is possible to heat up the body by the power of thought and breathing. If you can manage to charge your entire body with energy it's an incredible starting point for climax.

Anne's advice You'll probably find that your energy levels rise and fall. Don't be deflated by a fall – just go back to the part of the body where you lost focus and start again from there. If it helps, visualize the parts of the body where you're circulating air and touch them with your hands as you breathe. Then lift the hands away slightly and fan the area, as if you're helping the air circulate inside you.

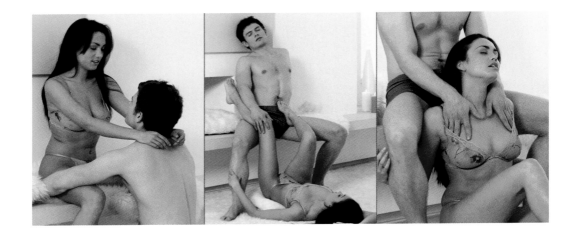

Pathway of loving intimacy

Having focused on the physical aspects of nurturing sexual spirituality, you can venture onto the pathway of intimacy and loving. This is a guided fantasy, which was introduced to me by massage therapist Kenneth Ray Stubbs (see p.219). It made such an impact on me that I've been unable to resist sharing it with others many times over.

FANTASY ISLANDS

However you choose to visualize your fantasy island, this exercise gives you a feeling of exploration. By sharing this fantasy with your lover and helping him expand his mind through the visualization of a landscape that intrigues him, you arouse his enthusiasm and sensuality. He gains a sense of closeness and intimacy from having experienced what almost seems like time travel in your presence, and it can provide a strong basis for some spiritually enriching sex.

It's best if you're sitting and your man's lying comfortably. You don't have to be undressed for the fantasy, although if you're intending to continue on to massage or lovemaking it's probably best to start with few clothes to minimize interruptions later. You then talk your man through the fantasy by outlining its bare bones. He equips this outline in his mind with his own scenery and embellishment. He doesn't tell you what he's seeing during the exercise but he can, of course, describe his mental images to you afterward.

> " WHICHEVER WAY A FANTASY ISLAND IS VISUALIZED IT LIFTS THE SENSE OF CREATIVITY. " *Anne*

PAUSE BETWEEN EACH INSTRUCTION:

1 "You are walking on an unknown shore. Picture the shore. What is its texture and color? What does it feel like to touch the sand?"

2 "Turn and face the sea. What color is it? What do the waves look like? Are they rough or are they smooth? Are they far away or is the water nearly reaching you?"

3 "Turn and face the beach. What do you see right at the back of the beach?"

4 Take your partner on a walk through the rest of the island, pausing always to get him to picture it and to feel the sensation of sand, warm hair, and humidity.

Anne's advice A guided fantasy is something that should be kept for very special occasions. If you try this too regularly the exercise loses its power. Practically any storyline will do, the secret is not to embellish it yourself – your partner's mind will fill in the necessary details.

MY OWN FANTASY ISLAND

My own experience of this was to see myself, not just on an island but on a different planet. The sand was purple and there were towering orange mountains nearby – a truly alien landscape. The trees and dense undergrowths were tropical and brilliantly colored, with exotic birds perched among them. As I walked through the forest, bright orange sand swept down from the mountains in rolling dunes, and soon I found myself in a hot desert. The fantasy was so extraordinary that it sharpened my senses and made my skin exceptionally sensitive afterward.

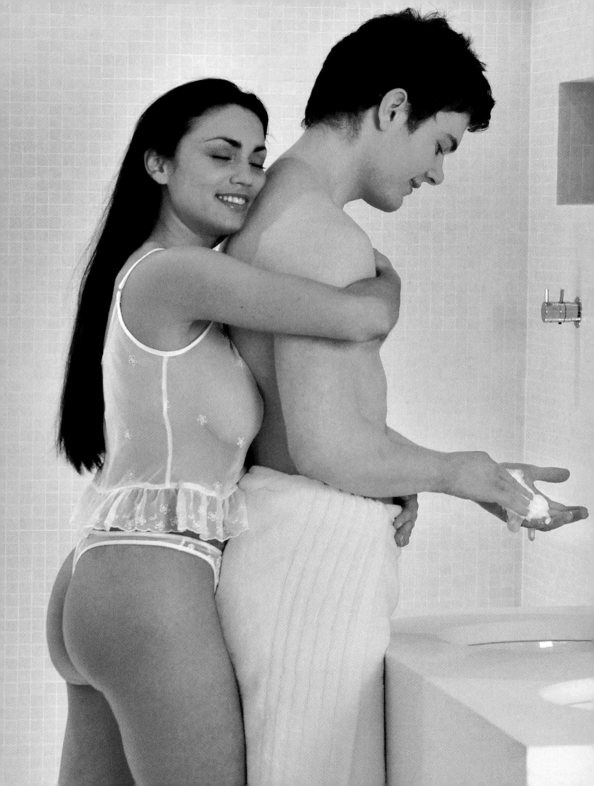

Trust and respect

Old-fashioned concepts of trust and respect are vital ingredients for creating a sense of spiritual peace between long-term partners. Many men and women possess a fragile self-confidence that can be easily knocked. They can be especially vulnerable during lovemaking.

LOVING INGREDIENTS

The ingredients that help build loving trust and respect are simple, but we often lose sight of them because we live in such a competitive world. Collectively, we've become paranoid, even with the partners we love. If you question this, try asking yourself if you:

- Always speak respectfully of your partner to others?
- Could think of five good things to say immediately about your partner?
- Feel like equals in bed?

MAKE **HIM** FEEL **TRUSTED** AND **RESPECTED**

Don't

- **Criticize** your partner to his face or behind his back to others.
- **Ignore** your partner's requests.
- **Lie** to him.

Do

- **Get more physical** with him and provide shows of affection.
- **Go in for hugging** – do a lot of it!
- **Tell him you love him** at least once a day.
- **Focus on him** at least 50 percent of the time. Don't just focus on yourself.
- **Be supportive** – in work, play, and health.

Therapy check Sex therapists know that when one partner wounds another with harsh words or sarcasm it inflicts mental wounds that affect subsequent sexual response. I believe the best sex takes place between partners who consciously trust and admire one another.

Ways to say "I love you"

Your man may make himself out to be tough, but he still needs to know he's loved. Sadly, many people find it very hard to say "I love you" or to demonstrate real affection. It doesn't mean that they don't love, but it makes it hard for their partners to tell whether they do or not. Assuring your partner he's loved is an essential – and easy – way of showing him how valuable he is to you.

GIVE OUT LOVING MESSAGES

1 Talk about the very early days of your relationship. Remind each other how strongly you felt love then. Then say, "I still love you very much now."

2 Touch, hug, or kiss each other in public.

3 When you watch television, sit next to each other on the sofa, touching and snuggling.

4 Care for one another's body. Personal grooming includes touch (see pp.62–63), and touch makes people feel loved.

5 Look each other in the eye – it's an extremely intimate thing to do.

6 Do three nice things for each other every day.

7 Make a telephone call every few days to simply say, "I'm thinking of you."

8 Read out loud to each other.

9 Always say thank you for things your partner does for you.

10 Every so often say how much you appreciate some characteristic of your partner's personality.

11 If you have to ask for some kind of change in behavior, include a mention of how much you value your partner.

" THE MALE WORSHIP RITUAL DOESN'T NECESSARILY HAVE TO LEAD TO ORGASM — THE INTENTION IS TO SHOW HIM HE'S LOVED. " *Anne*

Anne's advice Couples tend to learn from each other over time and there's a real chance that if you're open and loving, your partner will learn from you, albeit unconsciously. We can influence the people we are closest to just by virtue of being ourselves.

THE **MALE WORSHIP** RITUAL

Before you scream and run a mile from this politically incorrect notion, think about it for a moment. What if the boot were on the other foot? What if your man plainly adored your genitals — their very shape, touch, and appearance — and he showed this by bathing your labia, by brushing and grooming you, and by offering you a slow and deliberate genital massage followed by oral sex? And he did all this with absolutely no sign that he wanted anything in return — no pressure of any sort. Wouldn't this feel fantastic and wouldn't the fact that your man was so open about worshipping your sexuality make you feel pretty good about yourself? I know how I'd feel.

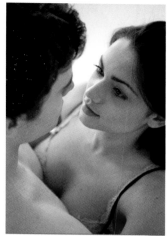

UNDIVIDED **ATTENTION**

If you want to generate fantastic feelings in your partner, who will worship you in return, here's a male worship ritual that you both might enjoy. Plan to do this within the space of a half to three-quarters of an hour:

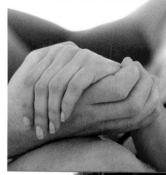

- **Undress** your partner.
- **Lead him** to a prepared bath and carefully shampoo him, including his genitals.
- **Towel him** dry with warm towels and settle him comfortably on a firm surface.
- **Massage** his body.
- **Caress** his genitals.
- **Tell him** how much you love his whole body, especially his penis and testicles.
- **End the session** by giving him an "oral massage" (see pp.118–133 for inspiration).

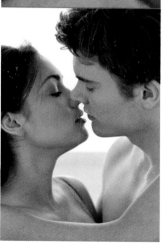

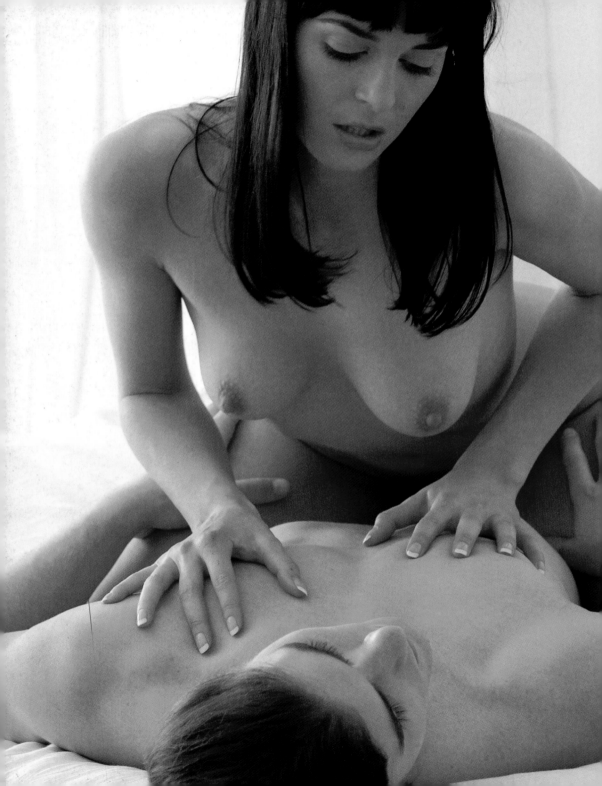

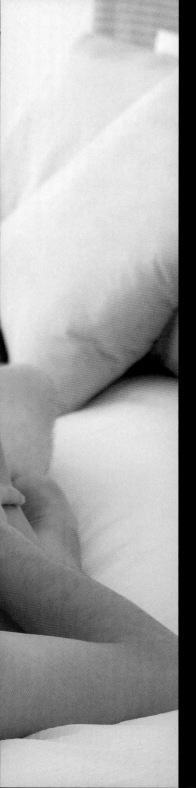

CHAPTER 9

Secret sex positions

Given a discreet opportunity, man
people would opt to watch anothe
couple making love, provided no
one knew about it of course! Mer
in particular, are interested in the
shapes and poses of sex, perhaps
because their acute visual senses
respond so stirringly to what they
see. This chapter will encourage yo
to become more sexually observan
and by learning how to increase yo
sensation during sex, your sexual
experiences will greatly intensify.

Triple XXX positions

lthough the great classic sex books, such as the *Kama Sutra*, list
ozens of sex positions, most of them — to be truthful — are either
ieant for fun only or are frankly impossible to imitate. It's clear to me
iat, although we adore looking at erotic acrobatics, we are rather less
·xually adventurous than we care to admit in the 21st century. Here's
iy selection of positions that are both adventurous and realistic.

·EW **SENSATIONS**

hese sex positions have been suggested for inclusion by
·e men and women I studied with on sex courses in San
·ancisco. The legs raised position (see pp.166–167) is
·commended; to him for deep penetration and to her because
·· can more easily reach her G-spot with his thrusting. The
·issors position (see pp.168–169) is a great one to try if
·u want to build up slowly to something new. The increased
·essure on both male and female pubic areas means that both
·· you will enjoy new sensations.
He'll love the grip (see pp.170–171) because he gets increased
·essure on his penis as you squeeze it between your thighs
·ile he's inside you, and back-to-front (see pp.172–173)
· recommended if you want to introduce some very different
·nsations into your lovemaking.

" HAVING AUTHORED
SEVEN EDITIONS OF
THE KAMA SUTRA,
I KNOW WHAT'S
WORTH TRYING AND
WHAT'S MEANT JUST
FOR FUN. " *Anne*

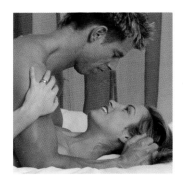

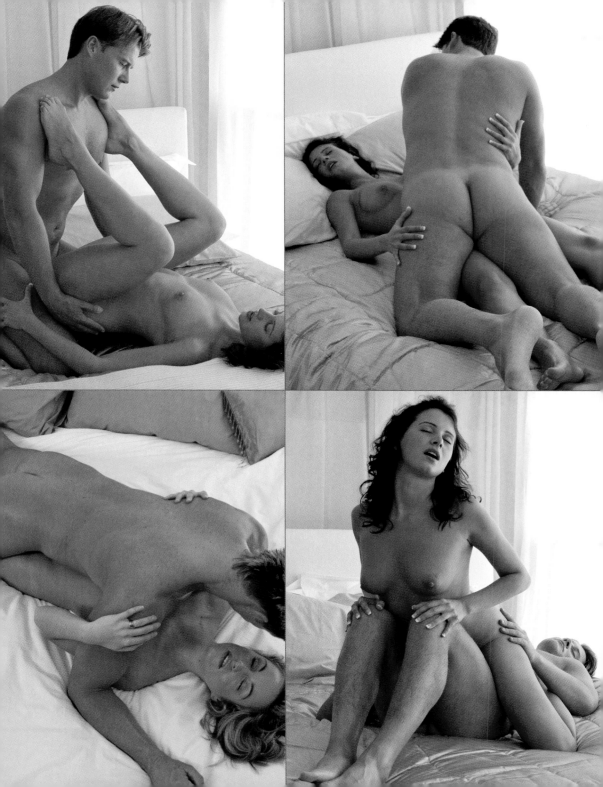

LEGS RAISED

This unusual position looks fairly acrobatic but it's easy to get into. He'll like it because you're so open to him and he can thrust deeply inside you. But there are hidden benefits for you. Your partner will probably find it harder to get highly aroused, which is useful if you want the action to last a little longer. And "legs raised" makes G-spot stimulation easier. Regular thrusting doesn't normally provide the intense and localized pressure necessary, but in this position he can lean back so that his penis is pressed firmly against the uppermost side of your vagina where the G-spot lies.

" THIS IS ESPECIALLY GOOD FOR PROLONGING SEX AND FOR STIMULATING THE G-SPOT. " Anne

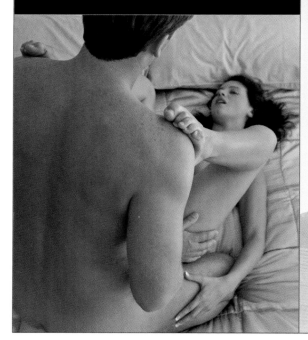

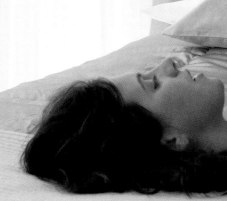

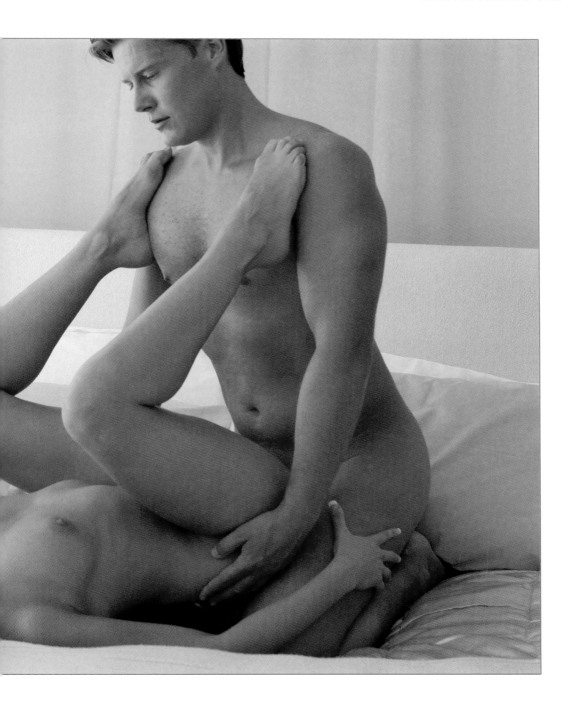

SCISSORS

This position allows for maximum pressure on both the male and female pubic areas. Seen from above, you make a kind of scissor shape with your partner. You lie on your back and your man is on top. But instead of lying stretched out along your body, he lies with one of his legs between one of yours and the other outside it. This alters the angle of the top half of his body so that, although your two abdomens are touching, he's actually lying to one side of you. This means that his arms are bearing some of the weight and he's not crushing you.

" YOUR TWO PELVISES ACT LIKE A KIND OF FULCRUM, ROCKING BACKWARD AND FORWARD ON EACH OTHER AS HE THRUSTS. " *Anne*

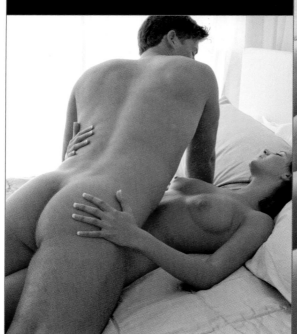

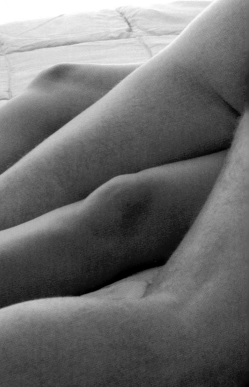

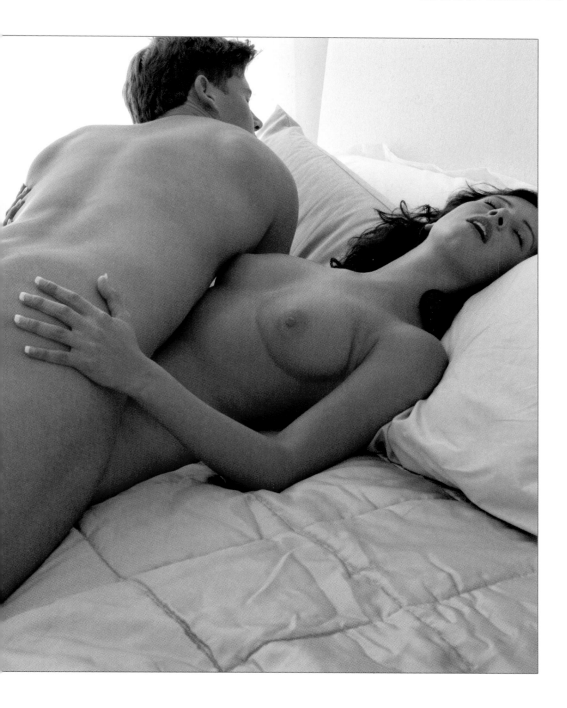

THE GRIP

As with the scissors position, you lie on your back and your lover lies on top of you. Once he's inside you, bring your legs together underneath him and squeeze your thighs together while simultaneously squeezing your vagina. He's now being gripped, not just by your vagina but also by your thighs. The sensation for him during thrusting is greatly enhanced because of the greater pressure on his penis. The grip's a good position if his erection isn't quite hard enough, and it's also a great help to the man who takes a long time to be stimulated to climax.

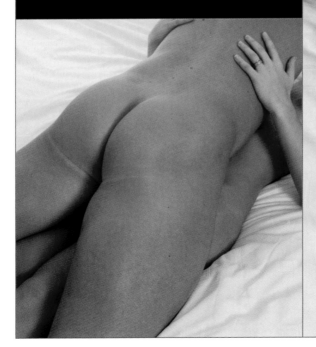

" TRY THIS POSITION IF YOUR MAN TAKES A LONG TIME TO REACH ORGASM. " Anne

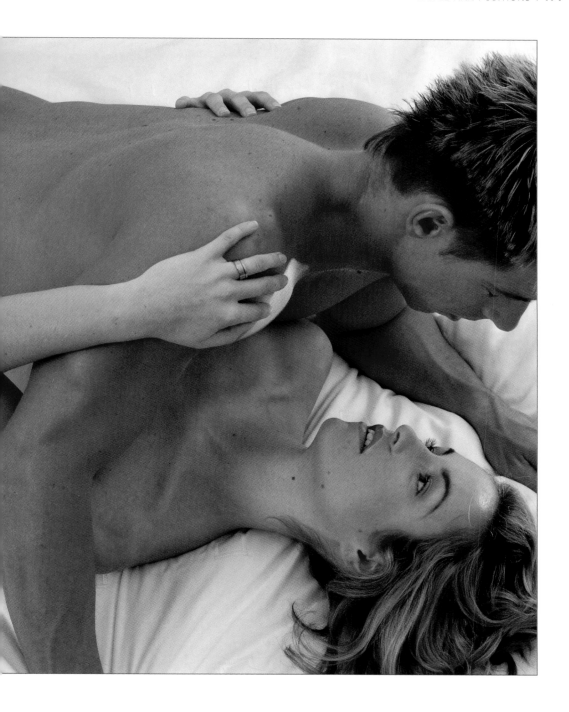

BACK-TO-FRONT

This is your turn on top while he lies on his back with his knees raised. Women-on-top positions are generally enthused about by men, who love to see their partners take control. This has extra appeal to him because he gets a first-rate view of your behind, which he can fondle at will. You can easily slip a hand between his legs and give his testicles some extra attention. The back-to-front position is really his treat as it's difficult for you to receive any extra clitoral stimulation.

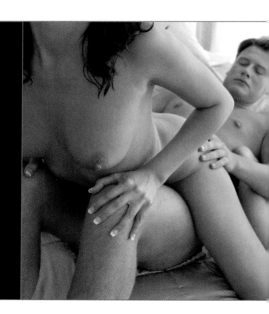

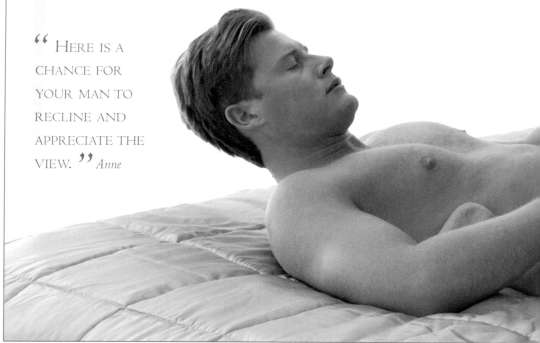

" HERE IS A CHANCE FOR YOUR MAN TO RECLINE AND APPRECIATE THE VIEW. " *Anne*

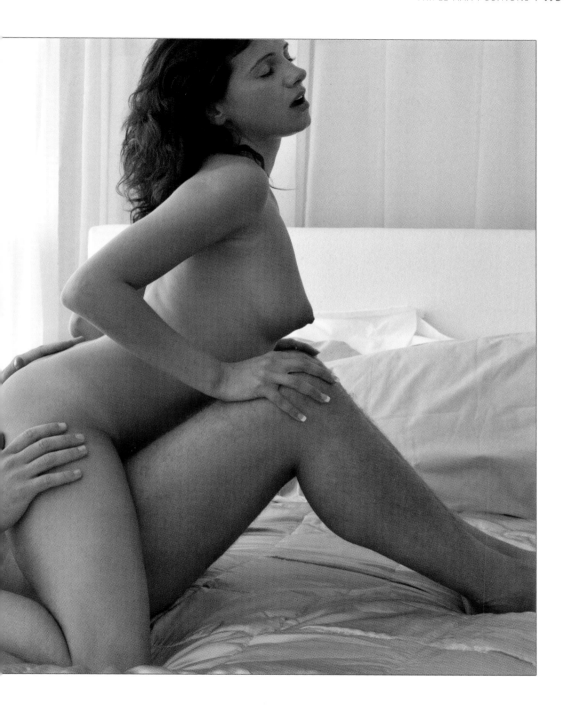

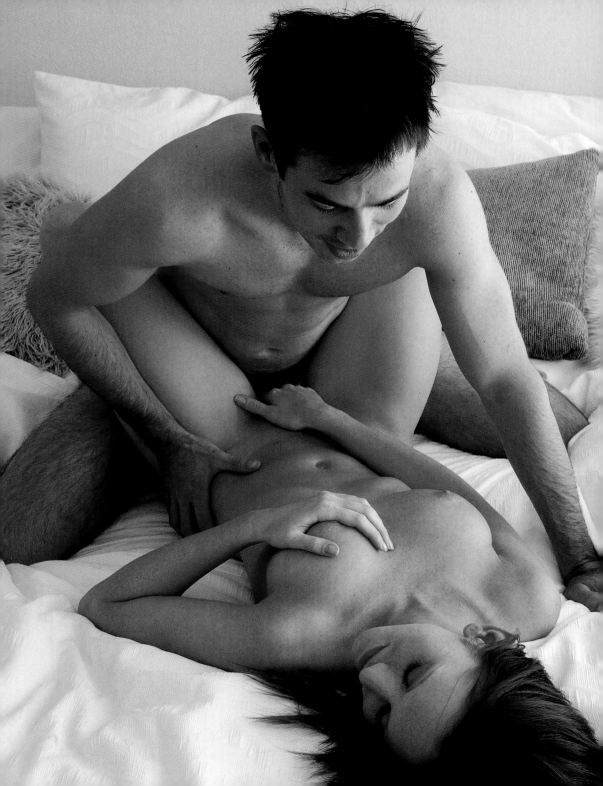

Secret variations

Many men can find it difficult not to come too quickly – and have borne the stigma of being labeled "premature ejaculators." One of the functional problems with intercourse is that if the man continues thrusting deeply he's likely to climax quickly. If a rapid climax is what you both want, then there's no problem. But most men, as well as women, feel cheated by having an orgasm so quickly – before they've had time to fully savor the special rituals and quirks that make sex such fun.

DELAYING TACTICS

Fortunately there are several ways in which men can delay climax (see pp.80–81). But many males want to be able to prolong intercourse without having to count or ask their partner to help them. In this case the flower in a vase position is worth considering.

In this man-on-top position his "stalk" remains within her "vase." He stops thrusting for a while as he continues to fill her up. Ideally, he continues to stimulate her using his fingers or a vibrator or, if this position is mainly for his pleasure, you stimulate yourself. You can use your fingers or try one of the mini-vibrators that fit neatly over the finger. They run on a tiny battery and are conveniently unobtrusive.

Once he feels more in control of his ejaculation, and when he can see that you are very aroused indeed, you can nudge him back into action. Should you desire simultaneous orgasm, this is an excellent way of achieving it.

Anne's advice Taoist sex educators specialize in teaching the art of delaying male orgasm. A key premise of their teaching is that you don't have to get stuck in the same position once sex has begun. There's nothing to stop you varying what you're doing as intercourse continues.

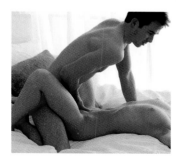

More fun on top

Your lover may adore you sitting above him and making all the moves in a woman-on-top position, but many women don't find it easy to get aroused when astride. In the rocking horse position (shown here), you lean forward as you slide down on your partner's penis and tilt backward as you rise up. This see-saw movement is designed to hit your particularly sensitive spots. By leaning forward and down, the base of his penis is more likely to slide up and along your clitoris, and by tilting backward and rising up, the head of his penis should bump right across your G-spot. Slow rocking also intensifies sensation during orgasm.

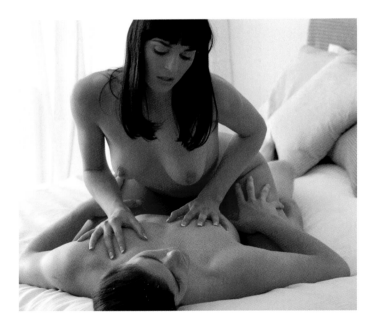

" YOU PAY YOUR PARTNER AN IMMENSE COMPLIMENT WHEN YOU GET TURNED ON BY HIM. " *Anne*

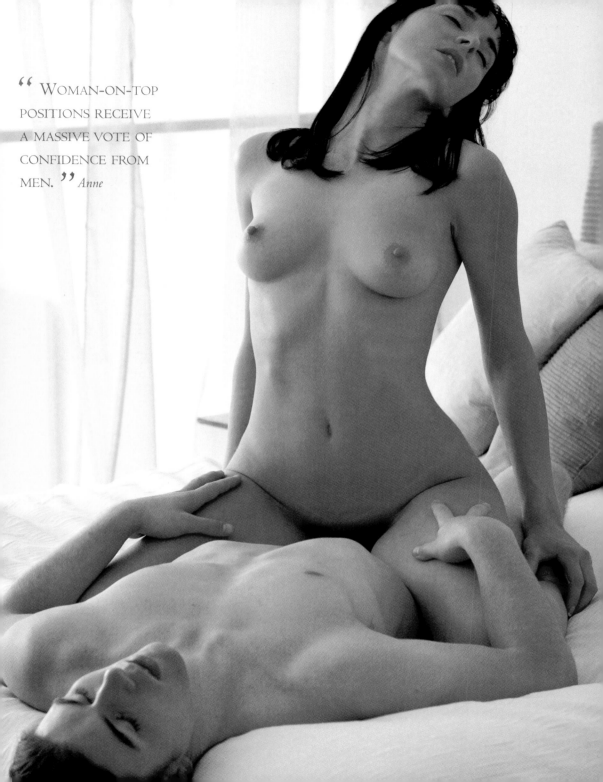

" WOMAN-ON-TOP
POSITIONS RECEIVE
A MASSIVE VOTE OF
CONFIDENCE FROM
MEN. " *Anne*

Secret strokes

My secret strokes are for men who want to experience their orgasms more fully. I use the ballroom dance rhythm "slow, slow, quick-quick, slow" as part of my sex workshop training for men. The rhythm provides a guide for men to alternate the speed of their thrusting so that they're moving their pelvis "slow, slow, quick-quick, slow." It can feel artificial at first, but the rhythm's so simple that very soon he forgets about keeping time and lets it happen naturally.

SLOW, SLOW, QUICK-QUICK, SLOW

This variation of thrust alters the pressure on the penis. Just when he's experienced the deep pressure of the slow moves, which give a lot of sensation, the quick, shallow ones delay imminent climax. All the time his sense of anticipation is building up. When he moves to the next set of slow moves, the sensation is even deeper.

There's a sense of timelessness about keeping rhythm like this that allows him to savor each level of sensuality as it builds. If your man's not too keen on this idea, it's possible for you to use these secret strokes on him in the woman-on-top position. This can get him comfortable with the idea and the new sensations so that he's ready to try it himself.

TAO "SETS OF NINE"

This is an ancient Chinese routine that was virtually unheard of in the western world until Tao ideas of sex were resurrected in the middle of the 20th century. It engenders great sensitivity in the male lover. Tao sex educators believe that just as the foot

> " SECRET STROKING CAN BE DONE IN ANY KIND OF SEX POSITION ALTHOUGH THE MISSIONARY TENDS TO BE THE BEST. " *Anne*

and the hand possess acupressure points that connect with other parts of the body, including the vital organs, so too do the penis and the vagina. In order to get the maximum health benefits from sexual intercourse, therefore, the penis and vagina need to be massaged thoroughly to activate the acupressure points. The "sets of nine" sequence is designed to achieve this and most of the internal organs are massaged in the process.

THE **SEQUENCE**
- Nine shallow strokes
- One deep stroke and eight shallow ones
- Two deep strokes and seven shallow ones
- Three deep strokes and six shallow ones
- Four deep strokes and five shallow ones
- Five deep strokes and four shallow ones
- Four deep strokes and five shallow ones
- Three deep strokes and six shallow ones
- Two deep strokes and seven shallow one
- One deep stroke and eight shallow ones
- Nine deep strokes

Like the "slow, slow, quick-quick, slow" exercise, opposite, the Tao sets of nine help the man last longer, but they also vary the sensation on his penis so that his excitement builds up slowly and thoroughly.

Men's reactions to it can be mixed. I know some who've disliked it because they've been so conscious of keeping count. But there are many others who felt it resulted in far deeper orgasms than they would ever have experienced normally.

Anne's advice A young man in my couple's workshop reported that his orgasm was very much delayed when he tried the "slow, slow, quick-quick, slow" routine and, that when it finally arrived, he felt it overtake his entire body.

Sex secrets "Deep rest" is a secret stroke for increasing sensation in any lovemaking position. As he thrusts deep into you, stop him for an instant and pull his buttocks toward you. Emotionally he feels submerged in sensation while you experience some pretty intense moments too.

Intensifying orgasms

These exercises form a part of Tantric sex training. They enable both sexes to slow down their orgasms to make them longer and sensationally stronger. It only takes a few practice sessions to significantly extend orgasm time. Reports are that the climax is likely to be slighter than normal at the start of the exercises, but much more intense by the end.

FLEX TO INCREASE HIS FEELING

1 First of all the man masturbates to orgasm and when he ejaculates he counts the contractions of his orgasm. This number is used as a base line.

2 On the next occasion he masturbates again to orgasm, but when he begins to ejaculate he clenches his penis as he might do if trying to stop the flow of urine.

3 He carries on masturbating very slowly while continuing to clench his penis, pushing himself on through the clenching sensation. If he can count the contractions again during this new experience he will almost certainly find that there are more of them, and the number increases as practice continues.

Anne's advice Try these exercises when you have plenty of time on your hands and don't need to climax urgently. Slow intercourse like this can be viewed as a kind of hobby reserved for special occasions.

INTENSIFYING A COUPLE'S CLIMAX

A similar technique can be used during intercourse. Use any method you like to reach the point where climax feels imminent (although a really slow sexual buildup is best). During orgasm the man flexes his penis and the woman contracts her vagina while they both dramatically slow down their thrusting movements. Practiced successfully, this can make the sexual experience so sensual that it's hard to tell when the orgasm begins and ends.

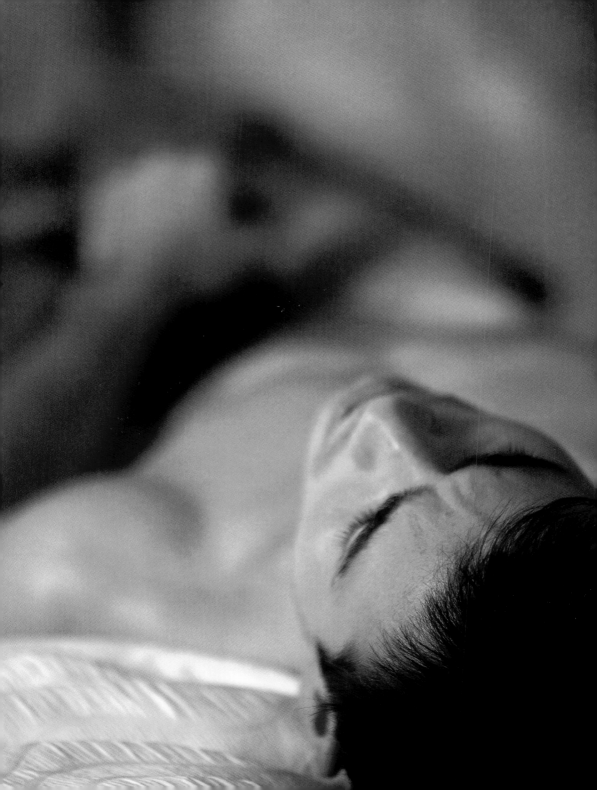

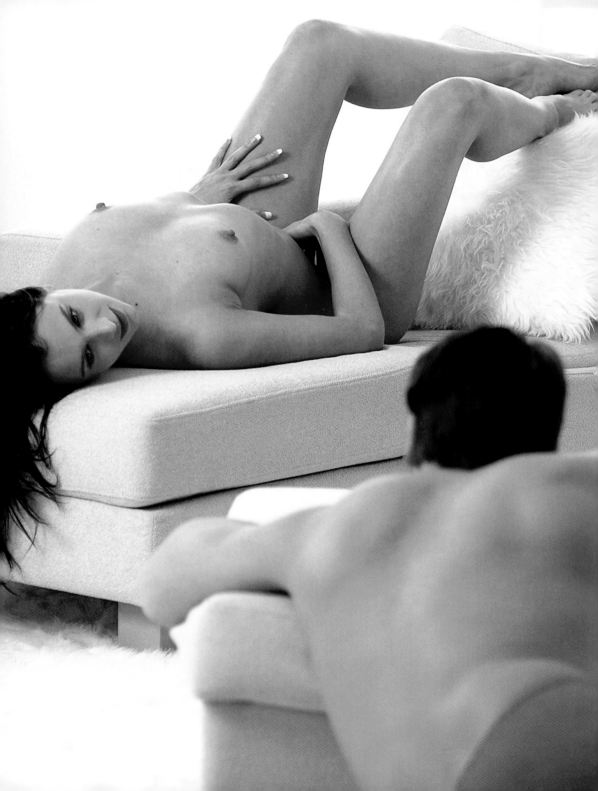

INTENSIFYING **YOUR** ORGASMS

Thirty years ago I ran the very first sexuality workshops for women in the UK based on methods learned from colleagues in the US. Before long I realized that each group tended to take on a distinct personality of its own and, if I provided the framework for discussion, the women could decide what it was they wanted to find out. I have since encouraged participants to provide answers for each other.

THE **ORGASMIC** FLOWER

One particular workshop group were very quick learners. Not only did they discover how to climax for the first time, they were soon ready for orgasmic fine-tuning. They weren't satisfied with just being able to climax, they wanted to have some of the best climaxes known to womankind. They discussed their particular experiences of climax and worked out some quite extraordinary refinements, including the orgasmic flower.

The orgasmic flower is a mental exercise that not only expands the mind, it expands and enhances climax too. It's a particularly female exercise and doesn't work for men. As excitement peaks, the woman imagines her genital sensitivity spreading out "like a flower's petals uncurling in the sunshine," as one workshop participant described it. This helps the woman to build up the final parts of her sexual arousal before spilling over into climax. If she continues with the visualization during climax, her orgasm is deepened and prolonged.

> " THE ORGASMIC FLOWER IS A MENTAL EXERCISE FOR ENHANCING CLIMAX. " *Anne*

Anne's advice It's possible to reach a point where you can dip in and out of orgasmic intensity at will. If you practice this during intercourse it can massively heighten the erotic sensations.

PERSONAL **ENDORSEMENT**

I was so impressed by the sound of this that I tried it for myself and I can vouch for it — it really does work. It takes your mind off the "stress" of aiming for climax and allows it to happen naturally. The minute you let your mind refocus on the physical climax you lose some of your orgasmic pleasure.

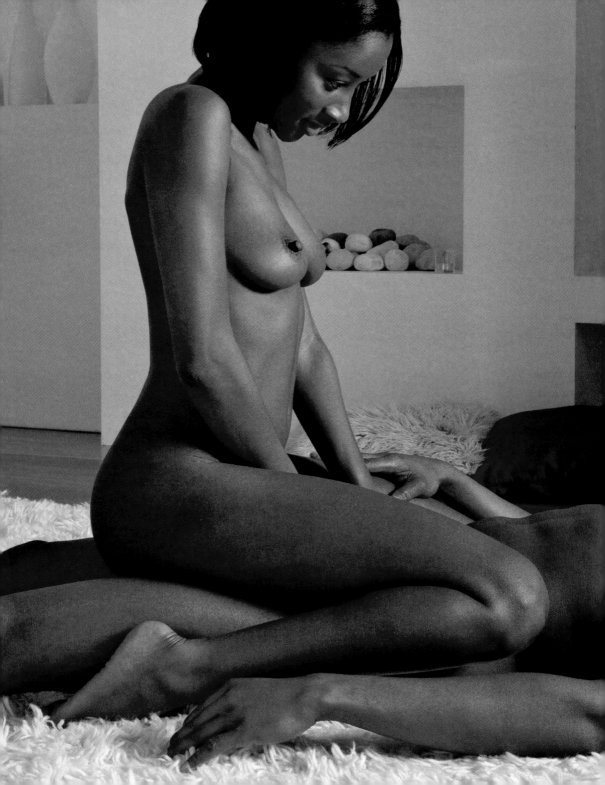

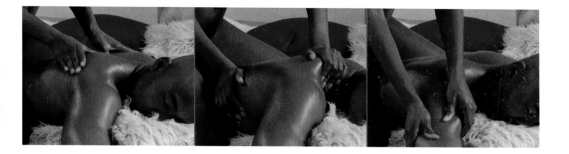

Climax all over

The famous US sex researchers, Masters and Johnson (see p.219), conducted some fascinating research into homosexuality in 1979. Among their findings was the absorbing fact that gay men often pleasured each other across the whole body for a very long time before going for orgasm. As a result of this long, sensitive buildup, their climaxes were longer and stronger than those typically experienced by heterosexual couples – who would do well to take note of these results!

WHOLE-BODY ORGASMS

The "climax all over" approach gives both men and women the opportunity to experience the sensation of orgasm throughout their bodies. Some women manage this spontaneously, but not many men can. You aim for a whole-body orgasm by pleasuring the genitals until the recipient is very close to climax, and then you go back to pleasuring the whole body. This ties in with the Masters and Johnson observation that arousal of the whole body using massage can greatly increase sensation during climax – the difference is that the genitals are massaged first.

> " DRAW OUT YOUR LOVER'S AROUSAL BECAUSE THE MORE EXCITEMENT HE BUILDS UP, THE GREATER HIS CLIMAX WHEN IT FINALLY ARRIVES. " *Anne*

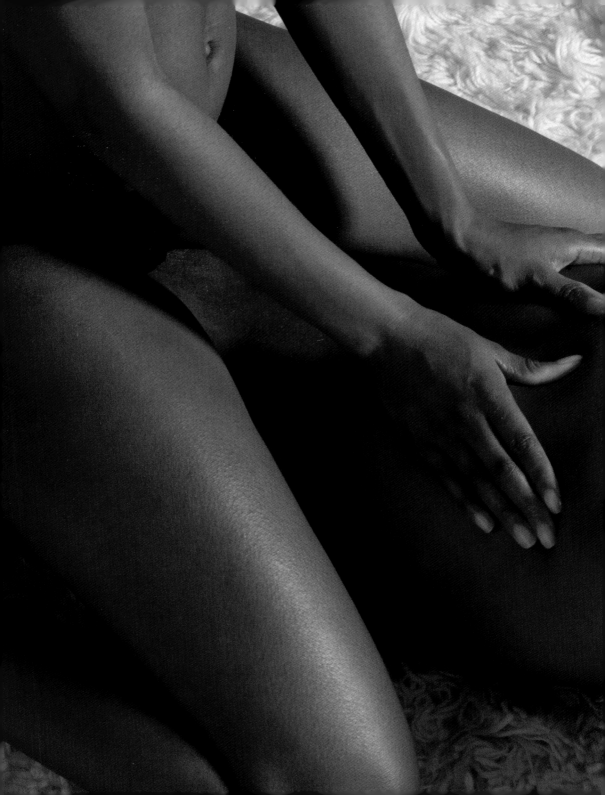

CHAPTER 10

Massage secrets

Physical touch shapes our moods and makes us feel valued. Perhaps the sensation of a loving caress reminds us of being carried securely in the womb, or of being cuddled and caressed by our parents. No wonder we crave physical proximity as we get older and custom prevents us from continuing closeness with our family. The massage secrets that follow in this chapter redress the balance by encouraging enduring expressions of physical love between you and your partner.

Begin with the best

You don't need to be intimate lovers to discover the wonderfully tactile art of massage. During my massage training in San Francisco, I discovered that if you massage a complete stranger you can end up with the warmest feelings of friendship and love for that person. Thirty years on I still have a special bond with some of the people I trained with because we shared an inner knowledge of each other.

THE **BEST STROKES**

Massage is of necessity a revealing experience – it involves bearing your body and rendering yourself vulnerable. This involves a high level of trust, and learning to trust is the basis of any great relationship, be it with a friend, lover, parent, or simply a massage partner.

You can't totally spoil your partner with a massage unless you put in the groundwork first. I've included here the very best of the basic massage strokes to get you started. These strokes resensitize the body, induce relaxation, and a promote a sense of trust. Once the body opens up, then so can the mind.

You can give an all-over body massage using "circling" alone – moving from the shoulders down to the buttocks and back up again. "Kneading" is a very good basic stroke for getting through to the deeper muscle layers of the lower back, hips, and buttocks. You might start "thumbing" on one buttock, taking it gradually all the way up the back and then doing the same on the other side. The recipient feels truly worked over and receptive to something a little sexier. "Feathering" is a playful and erotic stroke, best used after the main part of the massage.

Anne's advice Try varying the intensity of your massage by applying different pressures with your strokes. You could begin with a very firm pressure, then move onto a lighter touch, and finally apply the strokes with fingertips only, which can be very erotic.

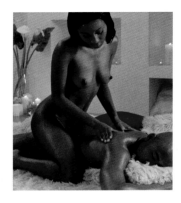

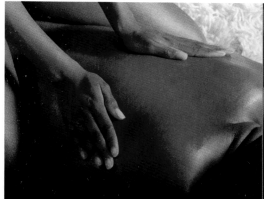

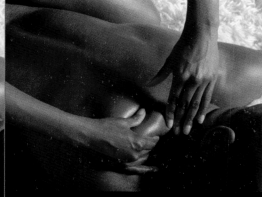

1 Circling Place your hands flat on your partner's back and move both hands out and away from each other in small circles. Circle them around like this repeatedly.

2 Kneading Using the thumb and fore-fingers of both hands simultaneously, rhythmically squeeze and release rolls of skin as if kneading dough.

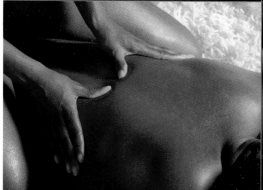

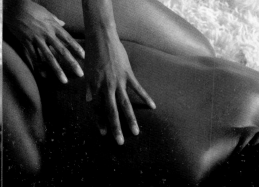

3 Thumbing Make short, rapid and alternate strokes with both thumbs, either in circles or by pushing them up against the skin for a few inches.

4 Feathering Lightly waft the fingertips of both hands in circles across your partner's body or in downward cascades of gentle touch. Be careful not to tickle.

MASSAGE GROUNDWORK

- **Create an atmosphere** in comfortable and attractive surroundings.
- **A clean, nude body** is best massaged slowly and leisurely.
- **For complete privacy** lock the door.
- **A massage table** is ideal, otherwise cover the floor with warm fluffy towels (a normal bed isn't firm enough).

- **Light some candles** and massage in candlelight only – as long as this gives you enough light.
- **Find a warm place** with no drafts.
- **Soft, warm hands** are best for relaxation
- **Warm some oil** in your hands first. Don't pour it directly onto the skin.
- **Try to keep an open mind** and ask for regular feedback.

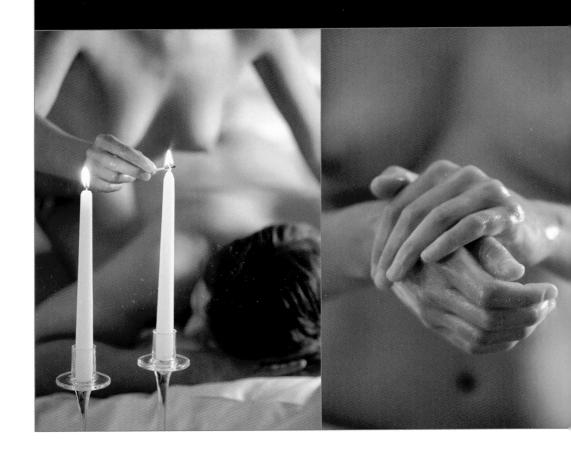

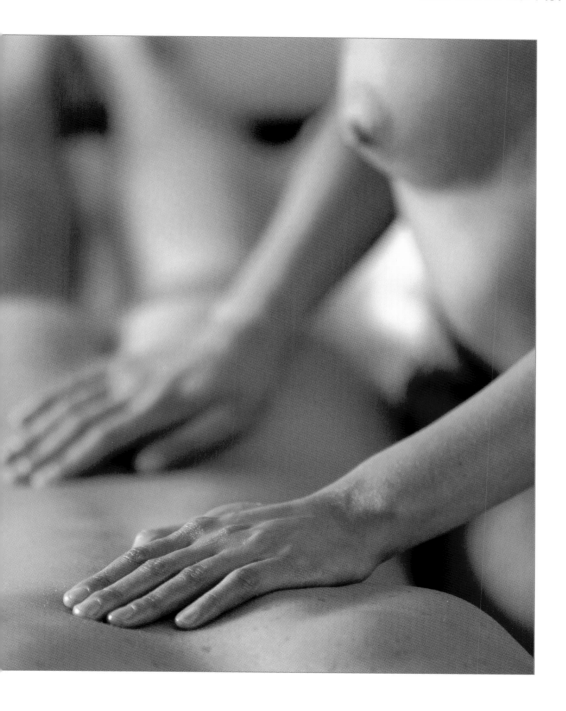

Male muscles

My lover of the past 30 years has wonderfully mobile skin. He's able to relax into a massage totally and my hands feel as though they instantly contact deep pleasure zones. It's not so easy to share the pleasures of massage with all men though because some males have rigid, solid skin, which is difficult to move. But by persevering and spending a little extra time it's possible to unblock tense muscular resistance.

MUSCULAR **ARMOR**

An explanation for muscular resistance was offered by a pupil of Sigmund Freud in Vienna named Wilhelm Reich in the middle of the 20th century. He developed a concept of "body armor," suggesting that some people are permanently tense and holding their body in "fight-or-flight" readiness. He argued that these people were unconsciously protecting themselves from the fearful outside world.

Massaging such individuals can be extremely difficult and some require deep tissue work of the kind that is best left to the professionals. But if your lover is tense, do your best to apply a really firm pressure so that he gets some sensation from your strokes. The more loving a massage he receives, the greater the chance he'll begin to relax. Don't be too downhearted if all he really wants are special "penile" strokes. Rejoice in the fact that he can at least enjoy fabulous sensations here.

" TIGHT MUSCLES IMPEDE SENSATION AND THIS MAY EXPLAIN WHY SOME MEN FOCUS ALL THEIR SENSUALITY ON THEIR PENIS, WHICH IS NOT ENCASED IN TENSE BODY ARMOR. " *Anne*

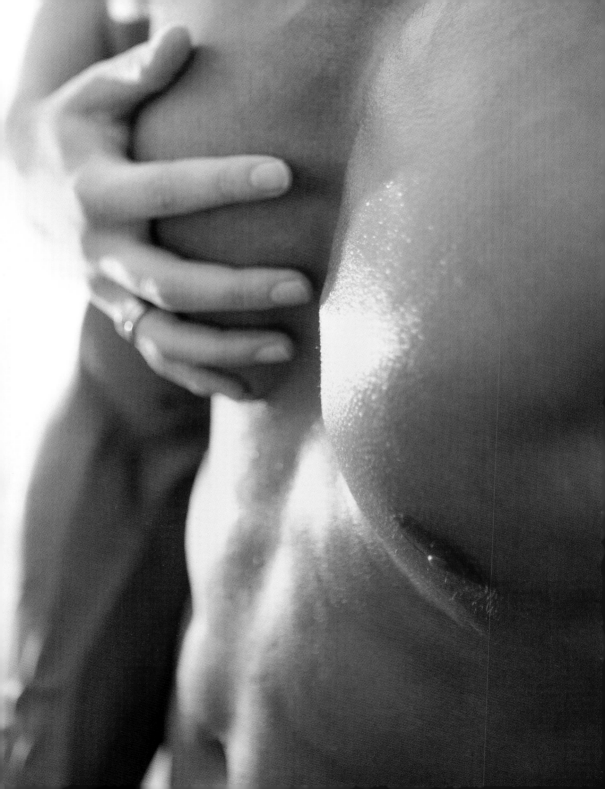

Special strokes

Some people feel sexy only when their skin is stimulated specifically, while the desires of others are sparked first by sights or thoughts, which then make the body more responsive to touch. These more advanced massage techniques are invaluable in both instances.

FOUR **TECHNIQUES**

- **Spinal tap** Place your thumbs in the grooves that run down either side of the spine. Press down deliberately (avoiding the spine), until you reach the bottom. Lean lightly on your thumbs and let the weight drive them back up to the base of the skull.
- **Inside the cave** Fold one of your partner's arms up across his back and lever the arm up slightly to lift the shoulder blade. Press the thumb of your other hand into the exposed hollow or "cave" and, still pressing, slide it out toward the armpit. Do this three or four times then repeat on the other shoulder blade.

Anne's advice If your partner's skin begins to go red, you may have been overdoing the attention paid to that particular spot. This is a sign you need to move on.

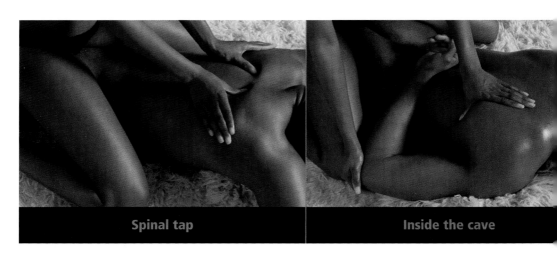

Spinal tap

Inside the cave

- **The glide** The glide is my favorite of the weighting strokes in which you lean the weight of your body on your hands as you are working on your partner's back. Sit across your partner's thighs and place your palms flat against the lower part of his buttocks, with your fingers pointing toward his shoulders and neck. Now lean forward, putting your weight on your hands and let your weight move your hands along his oiled back toward his head. You'll find that your hands move slowly to begin with but gather speed. As you get to his shoulders take your weight off your hands and bring your arms slowly back down his body.
- **The caterpillar** You actually massage on the spine when using this stroke, making it an exception (it's usually the muscles and other soft tissues that are massaged). Sit at your partner's side and place one hand at the base of his spine, fingers pointing toward the head. Place the other hand flat on top of the first. Next rock your hands backward and forward on the palm and fingers, allowing the bottom hand to do the pushing. With this backward-forward rocking movement, you work your way like a caterpillar all the way up the spine.

Sex secrets The skin can be thought of as the biggest sex organ of all. Underneath it lie thousands of nerve endings that send sensational messages to the brain when stimulated. It's entirely through the nerve connections between skin and brain that we get turned on – physically and emotionally.

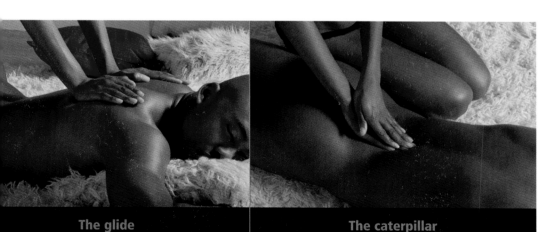

The glide

The caterpillar

CONNECTING STROKES

These massage strokes enhance the buildup to erotic massage. They connect erogenous zones at the top of the body with those at the bottom and, if they are made skillfully, the erotic anticipation can be very powerful.

- **Massage parts** of his upper body with one hand and his lower body with the other.
- **Marry up the ears** with the buttocks.
- **Pair the chest** with the inner thighs.
- **Don't forget** to connect the less obvious erogenous zones, such the back of the neck, the knees, armpits, palms of the hands, and soles of the feet.

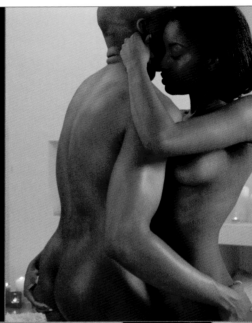

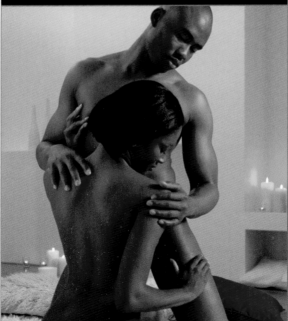

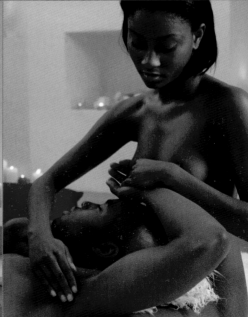

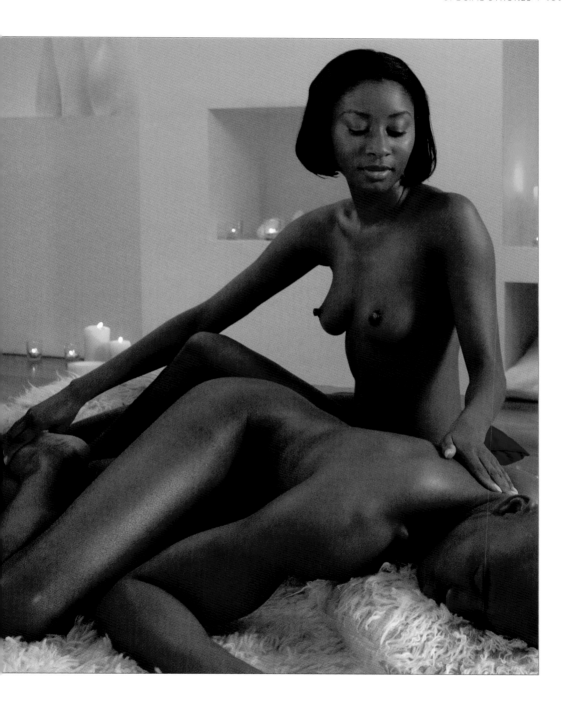

JOINING MOVES

When you've caressed your man into a state of yearning delight, you're ready to join his whole body up to the most sensual zone of all. Now you can deliberately link all the sexy parts of his body with his genitals. This will have the effect of transferring some of the excitement now raging in the far reaches of his anatomy directly to the penis and testicles.

Chest and genital strokes While your left hand is massaging the chest and nipples using circular strokes, move the right hand down to the genitals and make similar strokes along the penis. As you move your left hand to one side of his chest, move your right hand to the same side of the penis. You're trying to mirror the moves you're making higher up the body on the penis.

Finger and toe strokes Massage the palm of your partner's hand with one hand while letting your other hand massage its way down his body to his genitals where it circles around the base of the penis. Next massage one foot with the left hand and, letting the right hand massage its way up the same leg, gently massage the foot and genitals simultaneously. Repeat on the other side. Especially sexy foot strokes are those made on the big toe (see opposite).

The penis stroke Place the tips of your forefingers against the perineum (see pp.82–83). Slide the fingers up toward the penis, separating them to trace a pathway around the scrotum to the base of the penis. Bringing the fingers together, continue sliding your fingertips up the front of the penis to the top. Then slide your fingers over the top, part them slightly, and come down again on the other side of the penis. When you get to the bottom, separate your fingers out again and go back around the scrotum to the perineum. Repeat the movements continuously.

> " MASSAGE IS A FABULOUS EXPRESSION OF PHYSICAL LOVE — IT'S NO SURPRISE THAT WE CRAVE BEING CARESSED AND HELD BY OUR LOVERS. " *Anne*

Anne's advice You may have hinted at these joining moves throughout your massaging so far – your hands might have brushed against his genitals "by accident" while massaging his legs. This will have made his whole body yearn for the erotic attention you are now about to bestow.

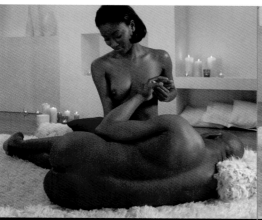

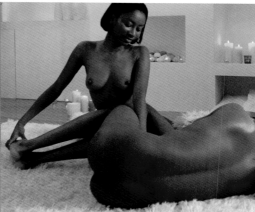

- **Lightly massage** the palm of his hand with one hand and reach down to his caress his genitals with the other.

- **Massage his foot** with one hand and reach up to caress to his genitals with the other. Repeat on the other foot.

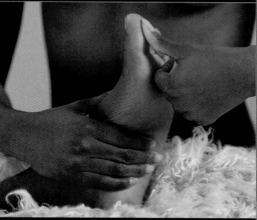

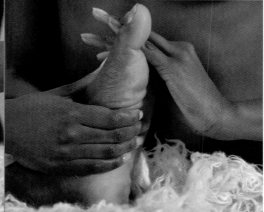

- **Circle his big toe** using your whole hand and then use very light touches to massage the pad of the toe.

- **Slip your oiled fingers** between his toes while sliding the fingers of the other hand around his testicles.

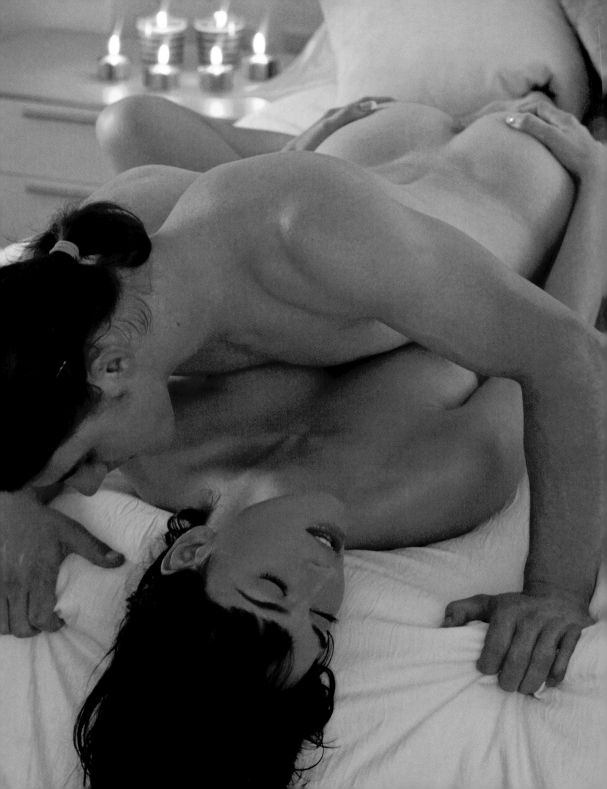

Closing well

Some massages are bound to end up as passionate sex sessions because of the way you introduce them. Similarly, the way you complete a massage sends powerful signals that affect the whole sensual experience. Yet just as it's a good idea to precede any genital massage by paying attention to the rest of the body, it's also wonderful to sometimes focus on touch for the sake of touch alone without any sexual aim in mind.

THREE-HANDED MASSAGE

If you're so incredibly turned on by all this massage that you can't resist crawling on top of your man, remember the ultimate connecting stroke. This is one where you massage him with your hands, while enclosing his penis with your vagina and simultaneously massaging him there. The aim is to make the entire massage, from beginning to three-handed end, a continuous flow of swirling tactile attention.

Anne's advice When I've experienced the energy sweep, I've felt relaxed and well as a result. You can feel your body lighten as a layer of energy is removed.

THE ENERGY SWEEP

Sometimes an orgasm is unwanted or inappropriate at the end of a massage, leaving the problem of how to disperse all the accumulated sexual energy. There is an incredible way to close your massage – by sweeping all the sexual sensation out of your body. Hold your hands flat, palms down, about an inch (2–3cm) above your partner's body. Imagine energy rising from his skin in great swirls – you may well feel this energy as heat. Make sweeping movements with both hands to disperse this energy along the limbs and out through the fingertips, toes, or head.

" YOU MAY NEED TO DISPERSE THE BUILD-UP OF SEXUAL ENERGY IF YOUR SENSUAL MASSAGE DOESN'T LEAD TO SEX. " *Anne*

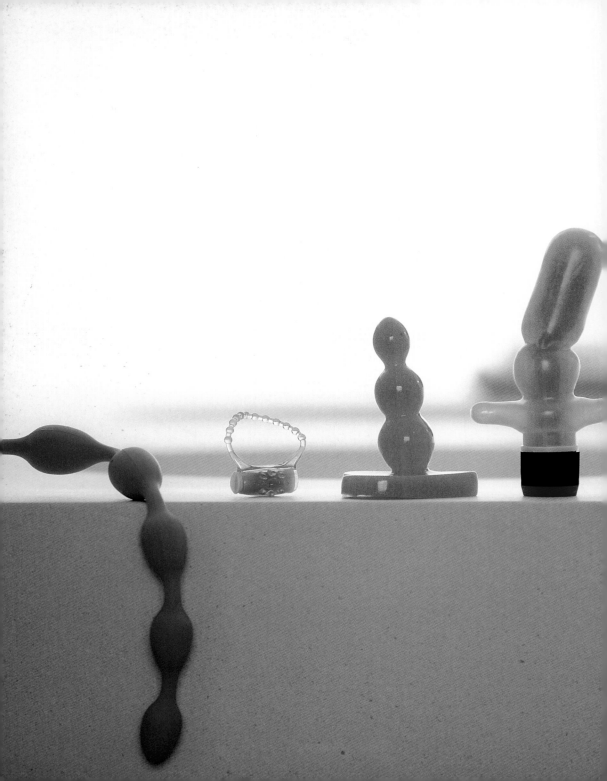

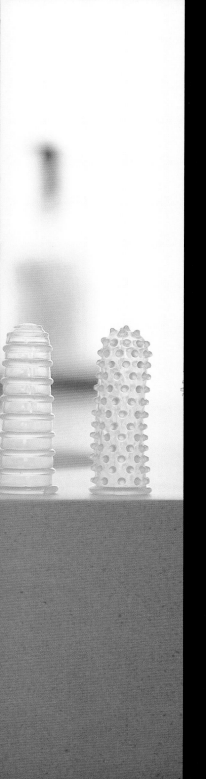

CHAPTER 11

Sexy shopping

Women feel more comfortable than ever buying sex toys, while men, of course, have been buying erotic aids and accessories for years. One result of this is that women often know what to buy for themselves, but are not so certain about what constitutes a good toy for their lover. This final chapter demystifies the best sex products for men and for couples. Here are the toys with classic appeal to men, but which will be acceptable nevertheless to you!

Best sex toys

There are hundreds of sex toys designed for men wanting to enjoy a sex life on their own, but here I describe some of the aids that are of special benefit to your man while the two of you make love together. Many of these toys incorporate extra design features that will offer you extra pleasure as well as your sensation-hungry lover.

EROTIC EVOLUTION

Although the colors, textures, and materials of sex toys have improved a hundred percent in recent years, the basic design of some items hasn't changed much for centuries. Women in ancient Greece used sex toys, as depicted in paintings on vases, and Roman men used dildos when suffering from impotence. It was the "uptight" Victorians who progressed the sex aid industry by making rubber dildos and clitoral stimulators.

COCK RINGS

These range from the spiky rubber type that slips down over the penis and grips it at the base, to the "stud" ring, or ligature, type. He can either slip a ring around the base of his penis (in front of his testicles) or place it lower down so that it's behind his testicles. The spiky rubber types of ring grip the penis and so help sustain an erection, while the spikes, knobbles, or other protuberances feel pretty good for the woman. With the ligature, you can pull the ring tighter so that it traps blood inside the penis. This is great if your man has problems keeping an erection, and if his erections are normal, it enables the wearer to remain outstandingly firm. Soft silicone rings can be stretched to fit any size of penis.

Anne's advice Your man should never wear a constricting ring for more than 20 minutes, and it should be taken off immediately if it begins to hurt. He should never use a cock ring if he has a circulation or nerve problem, if he is diabetic, or takes anticoagulant or blood-thinning medication, including aspirin.

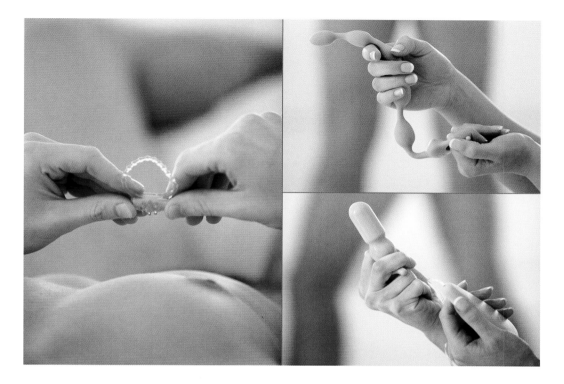

ANAL **VIBRATORS**

Vibrators designed especially for the anus are safe and stimulating. Both sexes can use them during masturbation and foreplay to experience wonderful waves of vibrations throughout the pelvic region. If you use one as part of foreplay before anal intercourse, it will have the extra benefit of relaxing the anal muscles ready for penetration.

ANAL **BEADS**

You and your partner may find these toys less intimidating than the anal vibrators and plugs, and so they're excellent news for those beginning to explore the novelties of anal stimulation. If you are able to pull them out quickly at the moment he climaxes, his orgasm sensations will be even greater.

" THE VERY FIRST STEAM-POWERED VIBRATOR WAS INVENTED BY A SUPER-IMAGINATIVE AMERICAN IN 1869. "

Anne

ANNE'S TRIPLE XXX SELECTION
From left to right:
• **Two anal vibrators** – similar to vaginal vibrators but smaller and with protuberances that restrict the depth of entry. One has a separate battery pack for "remote control."

• **Anal beads** – flexible elliptical shapes that stimulate his sensitive anus when pulled in and out. They can increase the sensation of a climax when pulled out quickly at the moment of orgasm.

• **Two butt plugs** – dildos for the anal passage that either of you – or both of

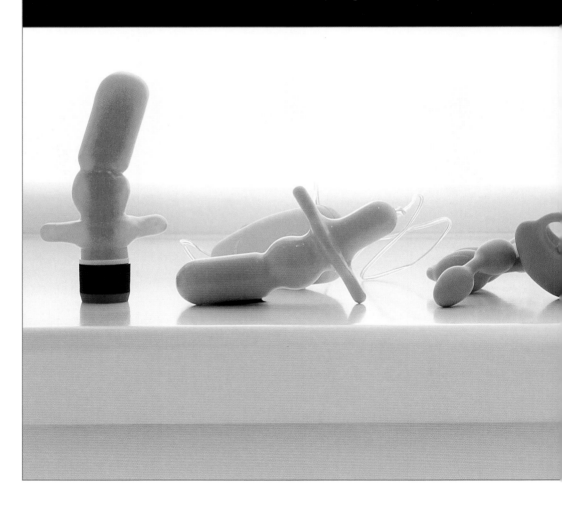

you – can wear for extra stimulation during lovemaking or masturbation One is curved to target the P-spot and both have a flat base for safety.

• **Cock ring** – a soft, spiky ring that sits around the base of the penis. Keeps him hard while stimulating your clitoris.

• **Two vibrating C-rings** – battery-filled sheaths with soft protruding spikes that stimulate the clitoris during face-to-face intercourse. The vibrations benefit both partners and are a must-try for women who have difficulty reaching orgasm.

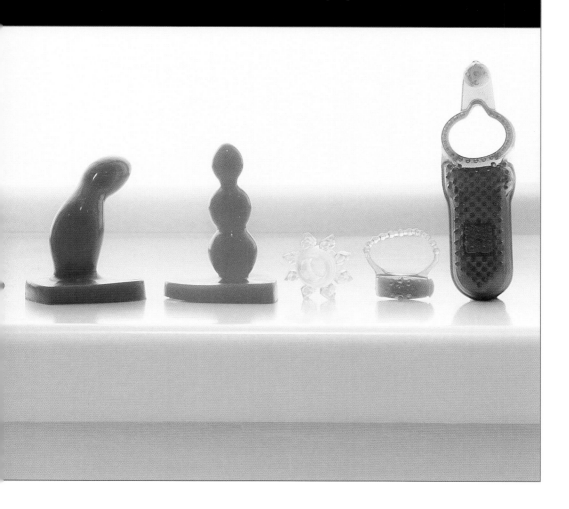

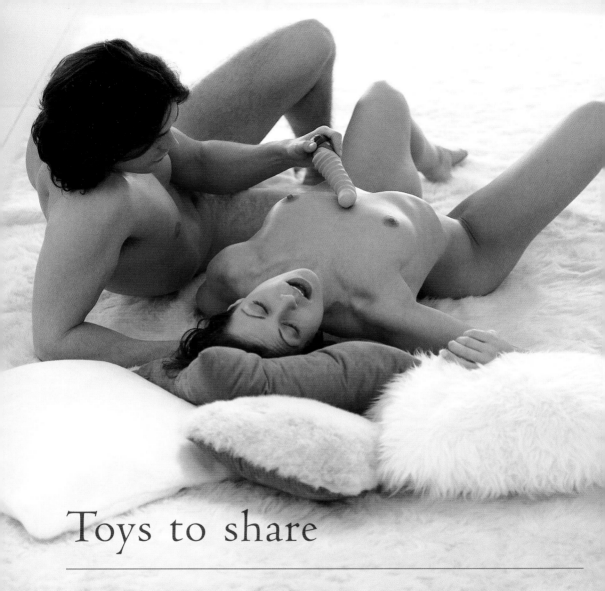

Toys to share

Today there's a real sense that sex toys have come of age. Not until
the end of the 20th century have sex toy manufacturers developed
specific toys for men and women wanting to use them together.
Enjoyed without shame by both sexes, these toys for mutual pleasure
are finally assuming their place in the market.

DOUBLE PLEASURE VIBRATORS

These toys aren't intended for use during intercourse but for mutual stimulation. They consist of two vibrators: one large and penis-shaped, which can be used for vaginal penetration; the second small and curved, which is used for his anal stimulation (the curve is there to ensure that the slightly bulbous tip reaches his P-spot, or prostate gland). The two vibrators are attached to each other and run off a battery. Some come without battery packs and run on a small bullet-type battery contained in the bottom of the larger vibrator. Most models have speed adjustors, which can be used to gain a number of different sensations.

THREE-IN-ONE VIBRATORS

These latex devices slip down over the man's penis. The top end (a rabbit-shaped tickler) stimulates her clitoris during intercourse, while the bottom end (a kind of raised bump) tucks into her anus. The toy is attached to a remote battery pack and, when the battery is on, the entire apparatus vibrates with the result that penis, clitoris, and anus are all excited at once.

SILICONE VIBRATORS

Made from user-friendly material that is nontoxic, odorless, and durable, this class of vibrator represents one of the latest innovations and uses of modern technology in the sex toy industry. Some older types of vibrator — and some modern ones from disreputable sources — can leach noxious substances into the skin, so do check the quality of the equipment you're buying. Silicone vibrators tend to be the most realistically penislike if you want your toy to look as close to the real thing as possible. State-of-the-art variations on this timeless toy include models that give off a sensual smell and those that are especially designed to stimulate your G-spot.

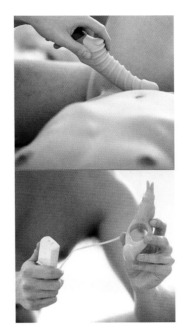

Anne's advice Never place a vibrator that has been used for anal stimulation in the vagina without washing the vibrator thoroughly first. Always clean vibrators, especially after mutual usage. If you're in a settled relationship with your lover and you normally have unprotected sex, you can safely share a double vibrator as long as you use it hygienically.

ANNE'S TRIPLE XXX COLLECTION
From left to right:
- **Two silicone vibrators** – nontoxic and odorless, these favorite vibrators provide maximum durability. They're light and easy to maneuver and waterproof so you can use them in the bath or shower.

- **Three-in-one vibrator** – slip it over his penis before sex and the "rabbit ears" will stimulate your clitoris while the "bump" will vibrate just inside your anus.
- **Double pleasure vibrator** – the larger vibrator is for your vagina and the small one is for his P-spot. These are

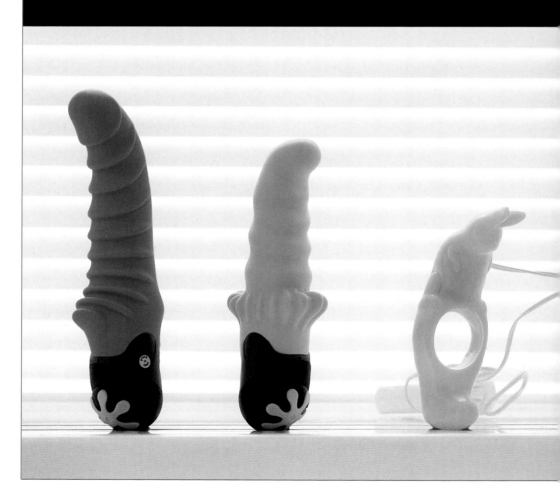

intended for mutual stimulation rather than for use during intercourse.

- **Silicone balls** – the latest version of this ancient classic, the two weighted spheres are designed to slip into your vagina for pleasure, alone or during intercourse. You can press against them to tone your vaginal muscles, which will increase his pleasure in the long run.

- **Double dildo** – these toys are made of a super-flexible material that enables both ends to be used at any angle. Hold the shorter end in your vagina and use your imagination with the other.

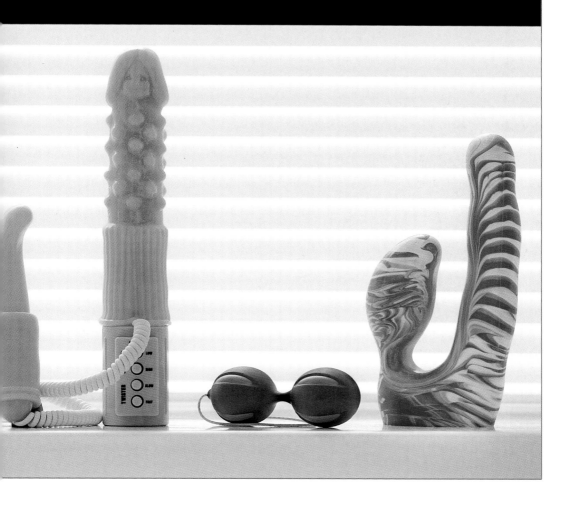

Expand his performance

Occasionally your lover may need something extra to assist him in his lovemaking. Happily there are modern aids that will expand the performance and satisfaction of both partners, and that won't make him feel inadequate in the way some of the older-style performance aids may have. Your partner may be willing, however, to wear a fun type of penis extension solely for your advantage rather than his.

TAKE YOUR PICK

- **Add-ons** Transparent, knobbled sleeves provide an extra 6–8cm (2–3 inches) in length when fitted on to the penis, specifically around the head. There are also skinlike extensions that may not look lifelike but can extend the penis by a similar amount and can also be trimmed to fit more precisely.
- **Edible lubes** These are small gelatin-filled capsules that flood your mouth with tasty edible gel when you bite on them. They are designed especially to facilitate oral sex. Bite on one just as you take your man into your mouth and he gets to feel flooded with sensation. You can also buy small pots of chocolate-flavored gel that you smear onto your lover so that you can then lick it off. Lubes should always be used warm as cold lubrication is about as exciting as cold soap.
- **Fun lubes** Cover your man's body with these good-enough-to-eat spreads. There are extensive ranges of them marketed in magically colored bottles. Their names reflect their exotic flavors — "mango," "red apple," and "wild blueberry." They're harmless if swallowed and, incidentally, sugar-free!

Anne's advice Don't make the mistake of thinking you're not functioning properly if you fail to manufacture natural vaginal secretion. Look at what is going on in your relationship before jumping to this conclusion. If you're not being adequately excited or stimulated it may be that you need much more personal attention from your lover rather than extra dollops of gel.

- **Natural lubes** Women, who for whatever reason feel they need a bit more lubrication to make intercourse more comfortable, can choose from a number of excellent "natural" products now readily available. Some of them are formulated to resemble natural vaginal secretions. They come in lighter versions for greater sensitivity and heavier versions for something more substantial, such as anal sex. There are also products made specifically for women nearing menopause.

The numerous brands of lubes in the shops are either water-, oil-, or silicone-based. Most are water-based, which makes them washable and harmless to condoms, but they can dry out. Check that oil- or silicone-based lubes won't destroy latex condoms or favorite sex toys.

" AN APPLICATION OF COLD LUBRICATION CAN BE A PASSION KILLER SO KEEP YOURS WARM. " Anne

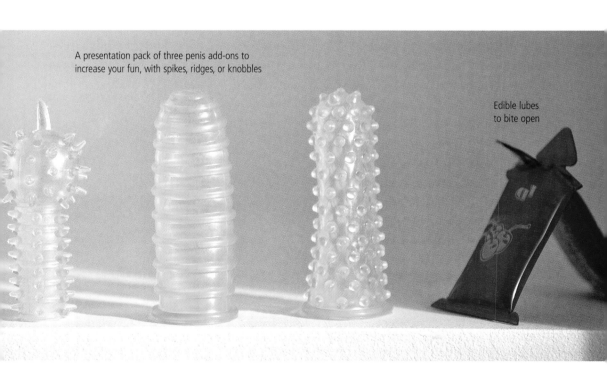

A presentation pack of three penis add-ons to increase your fun, with spikes, ridges, or knobbles

Edible lubes to bite open

Triple XXX erotica

Words and pictures about sex can be an immense turn on, which is why many sex toy catalogs advertise books as well. It's helpful to be aware of the difference between the sexes regarding the impact of erotica. Generally, women are turned on by what they read and men are turned on by what they see. The ideal erotica, to share between the two of you, would incorporate equal amounts of words and pictures.

SEXY **LITERATURE** TO **SHARE**

Many erotic books are timeless. The French author Anaïs Nin wrote collections of erotic short stories for a wealthy patron in the 1930s. Her titles, which include *Delta of Venus* and *Little Birds*, are still immensely popular. Women have been gripped by Nancy Friday's *My Secret Garden* since the 1970s. This is a collection of the sexual fantasies of real women. Nancy has since written *Forbidden Flowers*, *Women on Top*, and *Men in Love*. Violet Blue is writing modern erotic classics, including *Sweet Life: Erotic Fantasies for Couples*.

Men's taste in erotica is much more visually oriented and photographic work really gets their pulses racing. Popular modern titles for you both to enjoy include *The Fourth Body* (volumes 1–4) by Roy Stuart and *Stripped Naked* by Peter Gorman. The Erotic Print Society (www.eroticprints.org) publishes erotic literature, art, and photography. The *J. P. Smut* editions are quirky and nostalgic collections of the 1970s nudes made fashionable by photographers Jan Myrdal and Peter Smith. For some classic male titilation, tell him about *Crazy Babes*, a collection of 360 photographs by Bob Coulter.

> " SHOPS FULL OF PORN MAGS AND VIDEOS HAVE APPEALED TO MEN. THE BEST FUN IS TO BE HAD FROM EROTICA THAT APPEALS TO BOTH OF YOU. " *Anne*

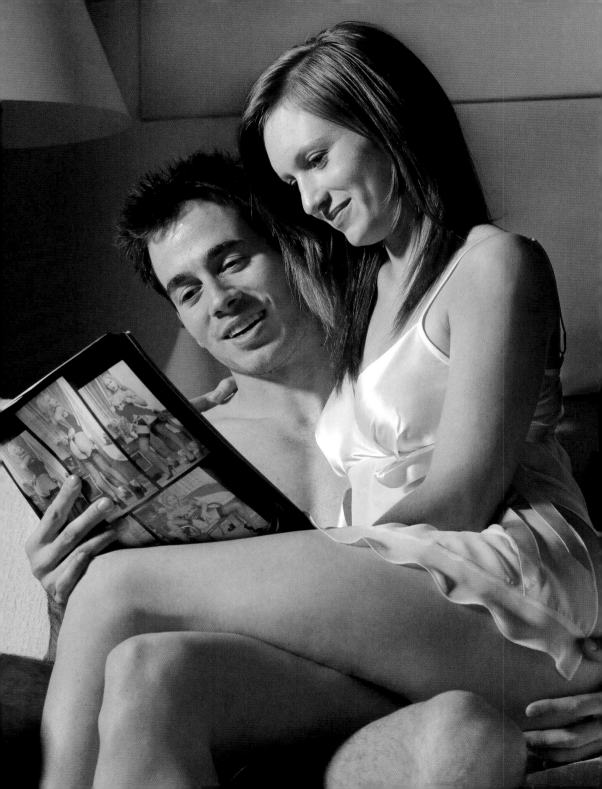

Playing it safe

Avoiding the issue of protection against HIV is not a viable choice for those pursuing an active sex life. Nevertheless we resent the interruption to the spontaneity of sex and feel embarrassed about handling the dreaded (but inevitable) conversation preceding the act. Here are some final pointers for safe sex without the mess or fuss.

REDUCING RISK

If you're going to protect yourself against HIV and other sexual infections, you need to be able to discuss the subject. An easy way to start this process is by getting comfortable with talking about easier aspects of sexuality. Tackle these slowly, using lighter topics first. Remember that self-disclosure is a good way of approaching difficult topics, such as HIV.

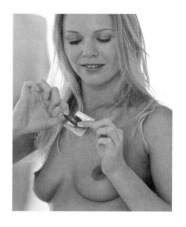

HOLDING THAT CONVERSATION

Try using phrases such as, "I feel very nervous about asking this question but it's something very important to me. What's your feeling about safe sex?" Or, "I know some people think it's tacky to carry condoms with them, but I think it's essential, don't you?" Alternatively, try asking the following: "I've often wondered about the value of an AIDS test. I can see how important it could be but I haven't had one yet, have you?"

SAYING NO IN A FRIENDLY STYLE

One possible outcome of a conversation about safe sex is that a partner refuses to use condoms or anything else that assists safe sex practice. Here's how you say "no" should this happen: "I like you immensely and I'd love to go to bed with you but

I really care about my health so, in the circumstances, I'm going to have to call it a day. I hope we can stay good friends."

USING **CONDOMS**

The good news is that many people these days are perfectly happy to use condoms, which offer good protection if used properly. See also pp.130–132 and www.condomania.com. This website can provide you with just about every example of safe-sex equipment you might think of.

USING A **DENTAL DAM**

Even female-orientated sex shops sell these now and the more you can fool around with them, the easier it gets to use them when the occasion demands. Familiarize yourself with the dam — it's just a sheet of latex that can be used as a barrier during oral sex. Show it to your friends and practice using it in front of the mirror having read the accompanying instructions carefully.

Experiment by using a dental dam on your arm. The aim is to get to feel so comfortable with the dam that your partner instantly feels comfortable too. This means he shouldn't have any problems accepting that you want to use it, and he might even look forward to a novel experience. It shouldn't be a novelty, of course, but rising rates of HIV infection among heterosexuals seem to show that it often is.

DON'T SHARE YOUR SEX **TOYS**

This is another important but overlooked aspect of safe sex. Although the HIV virus is fragile and dies as soon as it's exposed to air, it is possible to pass it onto a partner by sharing sex toys, such as a vibrator. If the vibrator were rapidly transferred from one lover to another, you might also be transferring the virus. Never swap sex toys without washing them scrupulously first.

Who's most at risk of HIV infection?

Highest risk activities:
- Unprotected vaginal intercourse
- Unprotected anal intercourse
- Unprotected fellatio, especially to climax
- Unprotected cunnilingus
- Unprotected anal licking
- Sharing penetrative sex aids, such as vibrators and dildos
- Inserting fingers or hands into the anus

Medium-low risk activities:
- Anal intercourse using a condom
- Vaginal intercourse using a condom
- A lovebite or scratching that breaks the skin
- Mouth-to-mouth kissing if either partner has bleeding gums or cold sores
- Cunnilingus using a latex barrier
- Fellatio using a condom
- Anal licking using a latex barrier

Great sex gurus

This role call of pioneers of sexual technique includes both academics and those who have led more controversial lives. They have all made us richer with their experiences and I have included their teachings and insights in this book alongside my own observations of the past 30 years.

VERA AND STEVE BODANSKY

The Bodanskys run courses on relationships, communication, and sex that are based on their own experiences. They have coauthored two books containing their research, and they demonstrate sexual techniques live on each other in their workshops.

BETTY DODSON

A successful erotic artist, Betty developed her "Bodysex Workshops" in New York in the 1970s. She made drawings of the genitalia of women in her classes and published these in her revolutionary book *Liberating Masturbation*, later entitled *Self Loving*. She went on to develop similar courses for men and is now regarded as a founding mother of sex therapy.

HARTMAN AND FITHIAN

Academic researchers Bill Hartman and Marilyn Fithian helped pioneer the study of human sexuality in the late 1960s and 1970s. They founded the Center for Marital and

Sexual Studies in Long Beach and jointly gathered invaluable information about the masturbatory and coital responses of men and women. *Any Man Can* (which describes the multi-orgasmic male), is perhaps their best-remembered work.

XAVIERA HOLLANDER

Xaviera spent her early years in a Japanese prison camp in Indonesia where her father worked as a psychiatrist. She was at one time New York's most successful "madam" and for many years she wrote the *Happy Hooker* columns for *Penthouse* magazine. Her first book, *The Happy Hooker* (published in 1971) sold more than 16 million copies.

ALFRED KINSEY AND THE KINSEY INSTITUTE

Kinsey and his colleagues gathered thousands of sex case histories and on the basis of these wrote two landmark books, *Sexual Behavior of the Human Male* (1948) and *Sexual Behavior in the Human Female* (1953). The books debunked commonly held myths about sexuality, including the belief that women were generally incapable of sexual response. The Kinsey Institute continues this research work today.

MASTERS AND JOHNSON

The acclaimed book *Human Sexual Response* was authored by Masters and Johnson and their pioneering research team in 1966. It was followed by several other books. The pair established a sex therapy program in St. Louis, which became a model for clinics elsewhere, and they trained other therapists. Masters and Johnson were married from 1971 to 1993.

LOU PAGET

Sex educator Lou Paget has drawn on fifteen years of research to conduct explicit "Sexuality Seminars" throughout the US, Canada, and Europe since 1993. She is resident in Los Angeles and is the author of several successful sex guides. Her advice appears frequently in the media.

ANNIE SPRINKLE

Annie Sprinkle is a prostitute/porn star turned performance artist/sexologist. She is based in San Francisco and has researched and explored sexuality in all its glorious and inglorious forms for 30 years. She has produced and starred in her own unique brand of sex films and photographic work. Annie also tours a one-woman show based on her life in the sex industry, and she presents workshops and lectures.

KENNETH RAY STUBBS

Kenneth, generally known as Ray, taught erotic massage at the Institute for the Advanced Study of Human Sexuality in San Francisco in the 1970s. In 1986 he founded *Secret Garden Publishing* to publish his massage methods, and he has since produced a continual stream of books and recordings. He emphasizes the sensual and spiritual connection between men and women as well as the sexual.

DIANE TORR

An interdisciplinary artist, curator, performer, and teacher, her installations, performances, and sound compositions have been presented in galleries and art studios throughout the US, Europe, and Japan. In Diane's solo performances she impersonates men, and she founded the "Drag King Workshops" in 1989.

BERNIE ZILBERGELD

As codirector of the Sex Therapy and Counseling Unit at the UCLA Medical School in San Francisco, Bernie Zilbergeld has practiced as a sex therapist and educator for more than 25 years and is one of the country's leading experts on male sexuality. His ground-breaking book *Male Sexuality* was the first to be written on the subject and it remains the best.

Useful contacts

SEX TOYS AND PRODUCTS

Anne Summers
www.annesummers.com
Mail-order or shop online for toys and accessories. Book a party in your home or check the web site for UK retail outlets.

Blowfish
www.blowfish.com
Supplier of thousands of sexuality and sensuality products in a complete online catalog.

Good Vibrations
www.goodvibes.com
603 Valencia Street (at 17th Street)
San Francisco, CA 94110
Tel. (+ US code) 415 522 5460
Email: customerservice@goodvibes.com
Toys and accessories and in-store workshops; two stores in San Francisco and one in Berkeley, US

Hustler Hollywood
www.hustlerhollywood.com
Shop online for toys, accessories, videos and DVDs. Check the web site for retail outlets in the US and UK.

Master U
www.master-u.co.uk
P.O. Box 32759, London SE1 7FJ
Tel. 08702 405737
Email: info@masteru.com
Mail-order leather and rubber bondage gear.

Skin Two
www.skintwo.com
Website for all fetish-related activites. Includes forums, online galleries, and events and clubbing guides.

Sh! Women's Erotic Emporium
www.sh-womenstore.com
57, Hoxton Square, London N1 6HD
Tel. (+ UK code) 020 7613 5458
Email: info@sh-womenstore.com
Fabulous toys and accessories for women. International mail-order service available.

EROTIC ART AND LITERATURE

Amazon
www.amazon.com
For an array of erotic titles check the erotica section of the Amazon web site.
These sexy e-book downloads are recommended: *Suddenly Sexy* by Jamie Joy Catto and *Office Slave* by J V McKenna

The Erotic Review
www.eps.org.uk
An excellent erotic magazine.

INFORMATION RESOURCES AND DISCUSSION FORUMS

After Glow
www.after-glow.com
Online magazine on love and sexuality.

Go Ask Alice
www.goaskalice.com
A US-based question and answer website for all aspects of sexual health and relationship issues.

Nerve magazine
www.nerve.com
Full-scale erotic discussion and personal anecdotes about sex.

THERAPY AND COUNSELLING

British Association for Sexual and Relationship Therapy
www.basrt.org.uk
Tel. (+ UK code) 020 8543 2707
Email: info@basrt.org.uk
Information on accredited therapists in the UK.

American Association of Sex Educators Counselors and Therapists
www.aasect.org
Tel. (+ UK code) 804 752 0026
Email: aasect@aasect.org
Information on accredited therapists in the US.

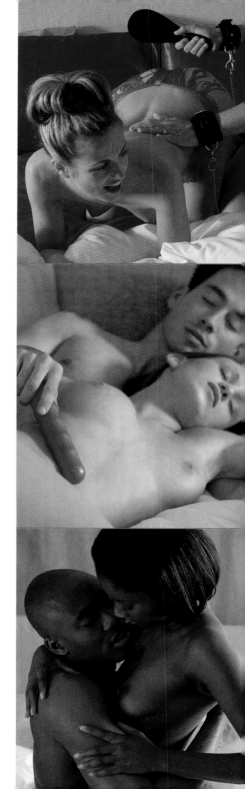

Index

ACKNOWLEDGMENTS

Photography
John Freeman would like to thank photographic
assistants Alex Dow and James Meakin, and
makeup artist Bettina Graham.

Illustrations
John Geary, Debbie Maizels, Howard Pemberton,
Richard Tibbits

Publisher's acknowlegments
Dorling Kindersley would like to thank Sh! Women's
Erotic Emporium for the supply of materials (contact
details on p.220), Constance Novis for proofreading,
and Richard Bird for the index.